THEOLOGICAL VOICES IN MEDICAL ETHICS

Theological Voices in Medical Ethics

Edited by

Allen Verhey *and* Stephen E. Lammers

A book from the Park Ridge Center
for the Study of Health, Faith, and Ethics

William B. Eerdmans Publishing Company
Grand Rapids, Michigan

Copyright © 1993 by the Park Ridge Center for the Study of Health, Faith, and Ethics

Published 1993 by Wm. B. Eerdmans Publishing Co.
255 Jefferson Ave. S.E., Grand Rapids, Michigan 49503
All rights reserved

Printed in the United States of America

Library of Congress Cataloging-in-Publication Data

Theological voices in medical ethics /
edited by Allen Verhey and Stephen E. Lammers.
p.   cm.
Includes bibliographical references.
ISBN 0-8028-0664-3 (pbk.)
1. Medical ethics. 2. Christian ethics. I. Verhey, Allen. II. Lammers, Stephen E.
R725.56.F35   1993

174'.2 — dc20   92-42800
                                                                 CIP

The essays collected in this volume first appeared during the years 1987-1992 in *Second Opinion,* the journal of the Park Ridge Center for the Study of Health, Faith, and Ethics.

The Park Ridge Center exists to explore the relationships among health, faith, and ethics. In its programs of research, publishing, and education, the Center gives special attention to the bearing of religious beliefs on questions that confront people as they search for health and encounter illness. It also seeks to contribute to ethical reflection on a wide range of health-related issues. In this work the Center collaborates with people from diverse religious communities, health care fields, academic disciplines, and cultures and disseminates its findings to those interested in health, religion, and ethics.

The Center is an independent, not-for-profit organization supported by subscribing members and by grants and gifts from foundations, corporations, and individuals. Additional information may be obtained by writing to the Park Ridge Center, 211 E. Ontario, Suite 800, Chicago, IL 60611.

CONTENTS

Foreword   vii
Laurence J. O'Connell

Acknowledgments   ix

Contributors   xi

INTRODUCTION
Rediscovering Religious Traditions
in Medical Ethics   1
Allen Verhey and Stephen E. Lammers

ON PAUL RAMSEY
A Covenant-Centered Ethic for Medicine   7
David H. Smith

ON JAMES M. GUSTAFSON
Can Medical Ethics Be Christian?   30
Allen Verhey

v

CONTENTS

ON STANLEY HAUERWAS
Theology, Medical Ethics, and the Church 57
Stephen E. Lammers

ON RICHARD McCORMICK
Reason and Faith in Post–Vatican II Catholic Ethics 78
Lisa Sowle Cahill

ON WILLIAM F. MAY
Corrected Vision for Medical Ethics 106
Gilbert Meilaender

ON JAMES F. CHILDRESS
Answering That of God in Every Person 127
Courtney S. Campbell

ON GERMAIN GRISEZ
Can Christian Ethics Give Answers? 157
James G. Hanink

ON IMMANUEL JAKOBOVITS
Bringing the Ancient Word to the Modern World 178
Marc A. Gellman

ON BERNARD HÄRING
Construing Medical Ethics Theologically 209
Ron P. Hamel

Medical Ethics and Theology:
The Accounting of the Generations 239
Martin E. Marty

FOREWORD

"YOU WILL recognize them by their fruits." So says Jesus Christ. "Action follows Being." So says Thomas Aquinas. "Walk your talk." Jesse Jackson brings the message of Jesus Christ and Thomas Aquinas to the streets of Chicago. Actions do speak louder than words. Our fundamental beliefs, values, and dispositions are revealed in what we do.

We at the Park Ridge Center analyze how action follows being in a very specific setting. In exploring the relationship of ethics and faith to health issues, we focus on how religious beliefs influence decisions about health and medicine. The very existence of the Park Ridge Center for the Study of Health, Faith, and Ethics reflects an interesting turn in the development of bioethics in the United States. It is a sign that bioethics has begun to double back to its original sources.

The appearance of bioethics as a discrete field is not a *creatio ex nihilo*. It is a mid-twentieth-century expression and expansion of a fundamentally theological enterprise. As Allen Verhey and Stephen Lammers underscore in their introduction, prominent theologians like Paul Ramsey, Richard McCormick, and Immanuel Jakobovits gave life to bioethics. Subsequent developments, though, virtually snuffed out the theological voice in bioethics. The richness of religious belief as a resource was sidelined by the conviction that our pluralistic society would be more receptive to secular discourse.

Recently, religion has found its way back into most bioethical discussion. It has gradually dawned upon many bioethicists that the secularization of the field was a mistake. Advocates of a secular bioethics abandoned powerful sources of insight and misjudged the centrality of religious beliefs and values to most Americans. In a nation where 87 percent of the people in a 1991 survey say that religious beliefs are important to them, it is hard to imagine that religious perspectives would not play a major role in shaping ethical attitudes toward issues in medicine and health care.

The rapid growth of the Park Ridge Center and the reappearance of religion as an audible voice in bioethics witness to the persistence of religious concerns in our secular society and provide access to wisdom we sorely need. The present volume may be viewed as a celebration, a homecoming for the distinctively theological voice that was lost to bioethics for almost twenty years.

Laurence J. O'Connell, President
The Park Ridge Center for the Study of Health, Faith, and Ethics

ACKNOWLEDGMENTS

By way of thanks . . .

Editors for volumes such as these have embarrassingly little to do.

We did have an idea some time ago. The idea was sustained and disciplined by conversations with colleagues and it became a project. Then many of those colleagues supported the project, first, by accepting our invitation to write an article for a series in *Second Opinion*, and finally, by updating and revising those articles to be included in this volume.

To say thank you to those colleagues is an embarrassingly little thing to do — but we should be still more embarrassed if we failed to do that little thing. We give thanks to and for our colleagues in this project.

Thanks are also due to the Park Ridge Center for its support of this project and to *Second Opinion* for running the series and for giving permission to reprint the essays. Sandy Pittman and Barbara Hofmaier of *Second Opinion* have been especially helpful and deserve both our praise and our gratitude. Their editorial and other assistance made the project an easy one.

Thanks as well to Eerdmans Publishing Company — and to our friend Jon Pott — for the willingness to publish these essays in one place and thus to make them more accessible to colleagues and students.

The volume is itself a reminder of what one generation of scholars owes to another, and we have been reminded of our own indebtedness to our teachers and to our students. Henry Stob and Bernard Cooke introduced us to the joys and rigors of theological reflection about the moral life and then held us to standards we only sometimes meet. And for the students who read what we assign and then challenge us about what it might mean, we are and will always be grateful. Without them we could not be teachers.

Come to think of it, without the regular question of students, "Where is this person coming from?" we might not have had that idea some time ago.

CONTRIBUTORS

LISA SOWLE CAHILL is Professor of Theology at Boston College. Among her many publications are *Between the Sexes: Toward a Christian Ethics of Sexuality* (Philadelphia: Fortress Press and Mahwah, N.J.: Paulist Press, 1985) and *Religion and Artificial Reproduction: An Inquiry into the Vatican Instruction on Human Life* (with Thomas A. Shannon; New York: Crossroad Publishing Company, 1988). She is President of the Catholic Theological Society of America.

COURTNEY S. CAMPBELL is Assistant Professor of Philosophy at Oregon State University, Corvallis, Oregon. He was formerly the associate for religious studies at the Hastings Center and editor of the *Hastings Center Report*. He has published a number of articles on medical ethics.

MARC A. GELLMAN is rabbi of Temple Beth Torah and a member of the faculty of Hebrew Union College. He is the author both of scholarly articles on medical ethics and Jewish theology and of modern midrashim for children. His *Does God Have a Big Toe? Stories about Stories in the Bible* (San Francisco, Calif.: Harper & Row, 1989) was named one of the best children's books of the year by *The New York Times*.

RON HAMEL is senior associate for Theology, Ethics, and Clinical Practice at the Park Ridge Center for the Study of Health, Faith, and Ethics.

He is a contributing editor of *Second Opinion*. He edited *Active Euthanasia, Religion, and the Public Debate*, a publication of the Park Ridge Center.

JAMES G. HANINK is Professor of Philosophy at Loyola Marymount University in Los Angeles, California. He is associate editor of *New Oxford Review* and contributing editor of *National Catholic Register*. He is currently working on a book entitled *A Personalist Vision*.

STEPHEN E. LAMMERS is the Helen P. Manson Professor of Religion at Lafayette College in Easton, Pennsylvania. He is the author of a number of articles in medical ethics. Along with Allen Verhey he is the editor of *On Moral Medicine: Theological Perspectives in Medical Ethics* (Grand Rapids, Mich.: Wm. B. Eerdmans Publishing Company, 1987).

MARTIN E. MARTY is the Fairfax M. Cone Distinguished Service Professor of the History of Modern Christianity at the University of Chicago. He is senior scholar in residence at the Park Ridge Center for the Study of Health, Faith, and Ethics. He also serves as editor of *Second Opinion*, as editor of the newsletter *Context*, and as coeditor of *Church History*. He has written over 40 books and many scholarly and popular articles.

GILBERT MEILAENDER is Professor of Religion at Oberlin College. Among his publications are *Friendship: A Study in Theological Ethics* (Notre Dame, Ind.: University of Notre Dame Press, 1981), *The Limits of Love* (University Park, Pa.: Pennsylvania State University Press, 1987), and *Faith and Faithfulness: Basic Themes in Christian Ethics* (Notre Dame, Ind.: University of Notre Dame Press, 1991).

DAVID H. SMITH is Professor of Religious Studies and Director of the Poynter Center for the Study of Ethics and American Institutions at Indiana University in Bloomington. He has written *Health and Medicine in the Anglican Tradition: Conscience, Community and Compromise* (New York: Crossroad Publishing Company, 1986). He is currently working on a book entitled *How Firm a Foundation: Religion and Medical Ethics*.

ALLEN VERHEY is the Director and Research Fellow at the Institute of Religion at the Texas Medical Center in Houston, Texas. Along with

Contributors

Stephen Lammers he is the editor of *On Moral Medicine: Theological Perspectives on Medical Ethics* (Grand Rapids, Mich.: Wm. B. Eerdmans Publishing Company, 1987). He is coauthor of *Christian Faith, Health, and Medical Practice* (Grand Rapids, Mich.: Wm. B. Eerdmans Publishing Company, 1989).

INTRODUCTION

Rediscovering Religious Traditions in Medical Ethics

ALLEN VERHEY *and* STEPHEN E. LAMMERS

DANIEL Callahan — one of the first moral philosophers to become interested in medical ethics and still one of the finest — has provided "a short history of bioethics." That history, abridged and amended here, may serve as an introduction to this collection of essays on the contributions of theologians to medical ethics.

Callahan's "short history" traces the beginnings of modern medical ethics as a distinctive field of inquiry to the 1954 book by Joseph Fletcher, *Medicine and Morals*, but he acknowledges that the explosion of interest came more than a decade later. In the middle of the sixties public attention was drawn to a series of hard moral questions about medicine — questions about experimentation and the protection of human subjects, about transplants and the definition of death, about prenatal diagnosis and genetic counseling, about kidney dialysis and the allocation of scarce medical resources — and bioethics was born.

The questions seemed novel, but there were some resources and traditions for reasonable reflection and responsible action in answer to them. Callahan reports that most of the resources were found in religious traditions; as he acknowledges autobiographically, "When I first became interested in bioethics in the mid-1960's, the only resources were theological or those drawn from within the traditions of medicine, themselves heavily shaped by religion" (1990: 2). It is little wonder, then,

1

INTRODUCTION

that in what Callahan calls "the emergence of the field" (1990: 3) —
and in what another scholar calls "the renaissance of medical ethics"
(Walters 1985) — theologians were to play a major role.

Bioethics may have a "short history," but the religious traditions
of reflection about the ordinary human events of giving birth and
suffering and dying are long and worthy ones. For centuries, Christians,
Jews, and other religious people have tried to interpret those events and
to respond to them in ways appropriate to their convictions about God
and the cause of God. There was plenty of foolishness mixed in with
the wisdom of those traditions, of course, but the traditions were there.
The traditions were resources for doctors and nurses who tried con-
scientiously to bring their practice into line with their religious profession. The traditions were resources for patients who tried to make
decisions about medical care that would be faithful to their religious
convictions and loyalties. The traditions were resources for ministers
and other religious leaders who struggled to discern the words and deeds
that would appropriately encourage or admonish a medical professional
or a patient. And the traditions were resources for those in the middle
of the 1960s who began to consider the extraordinary new powers of
medicine and the new moral problems they posed.

Some of the most significant theological voices in those early
conversations about medical ethics are treated in this volume. Callahan's
"short history" calls attention to Paul Ramsey, who — always writing,
to take him at his word, as "a Christian ethicist, and not as some
hypothetical common denominator" (Ramsey 1974: 56) — opened up
this new field of inquiry with his "explorations into medical ethics" in
The Patient as Person (Ramsey 1970). Callahan also mentions James
Gustafson, another Protestant and another compelling theological voice,
and Richard McCormick, a Roman Catholic who probed and utilized
that tradition. Immanuel Jakobovits had written *Jewish Medical Ethics*
(1959) a decade earlier, and that text provided a resource and a model
for other Jewish voices in the emergence of medical ethics. Other Protestants, like Stanley Hauerwas and William May and James Childress,
and other Catholics, like Germain Grisez and Bernard Häring, soon
joined their voices to the discussion.

And others, too, not treated in this volume, contributed to the
debate. A list of other early Protestant contributors would include,
among others, Arthur Dyck, John Fletcher, Joseph Fletcher, J. Robert
Nelson, Gene Outka, Ralph Potter, David H. Smith (who contributes

2

the essay on Ramsey to this volume), Harmon Smith, Kenneth Vaux, Robert Veatch, and LeRoy Walters. A list of early Roman Catholic contributors would include, among others, John Connery, Charles Curran, Albert Jonsen, Dan Maguire, William E. May, Edmund Pellegrino, and Warren Reich. And a list of other early Jewish contributors would include, again among others, J. David Bleich, David Feldman, Ronald Green, David Novak, Fred Rosner, and Seymour Siegel. Each in his own way worked to rediscover the religious tradition about issues of medical care and to make it useful to the emerging field. The retrieval of tradition was always selective, and there was frequently tension between the demands for continuity and the demands for change, both of which belong to fidelity to a tradition. Theologians — and the religious traditions they rediscovered — played an important role in the emergence of the field of modern medical ethics.

However, as Callahan's "short history" makes clear, after the "renaissance of medical ethics" came the "enlightenment" of medical ethics. In the next decade, interest in religious traditions moved from the center to the margins of scholarly attention in medical ethics. The theologians who continued to contribute to the field seldom made an explicit appeal to their theological convictions or to their religious traditions. Callahan identifies a number of reasons for this, but chief among them was the conviction emerging within the field that public debate about medical ethics in a pluralistic society would be best served by the application of "an ethic of universal principles — especially autonomy, beneficence, and justice" (Callahan 1990: 3).

That is the model and those are the principles given pride of place in the 1978 *Belmont Report* of the National Commission for the Protection of Human Subjects. And that is the model and those are the principles accepted also by some of the theologians who worked in medical ethics during this period. Of course, one could give theological backing for such a model and such a project for medical ethics. And, of course, some theologians raised their voice in protest against the "secularization" of medical ethics. The reader of this volume might compare, for example, the work of James Childress and Stanley Hauerwas as responses to the "enlightenment" of medical ethics. At any rate, there was, and continues to be, an enlightenment suspicion of particular traditions and an enlightenment celebration of individual autonomy over against the "authority" of priest and magistrate and that new figure of arbitrary dominance, the physician. The importance of an arena of "privacy," a space for autonomy and preference, was and is underscored, but it was and is also underscored that what matters publicly is simply that there should be such a space, not how it is filled. Religious convictions and particular traditions were and are assigned to that private space, and so to the margins of the public discourse and debate.

But Callahan's "short history" does not end there. At the end of his article he calls attention to what he calls "the discontents of secularization" (Callahan 1990: 4). He acknowledges that the muting of religious voices has been costly to the field and to public discourse. He identifies three costs: The debates about medical ethics have grown "too heavily dependent upon the law as the working source of morality," have been "bereft of the accumulated wisdom and knowledge that are the fruit of long-established religious traditions," and have been "forced to pretend that we are not creatures . . . of particular communities" (Callahan 1990: 4). The "short history" points toward a future for the field in which religious voices may and should have a significant role again.

Callahan's "discontents with secularization" and his invitation to rediscover again religious traditions for medical ethics and to give them voice again are particularly poignant. The essay is powerfully personal. Callahan reports that he had been "through much of the 1960's a religious person," but that he no longer regards himself as a believer. He can no longer speak in a religious voice himself. But he recognizes that the efforts to speak a universal moral language, what Jeffrey Stout calls "moral esperanto" (Stout 1988: 60-81, 294), reduce morality to the set of minimal expectations necessary for pluralism, and that they "enshrine the discourse of wary strangers (especially that of rights) as the preferred mode of daily relations" (Callahan 1990: 4).

Perhaps, as Alasdair MacIntyre claims, the enlightenment project has failed (MacIntyre 1981: 49-75); but even if it has not altogether failed, Callahan would remind us not to be pretentious about its successes. One need not deny that there are some minimal moral standards that can be defended rationally to a universal audience in order to recognize that such standards do and can provide only a minimal account of what is morally at stake in medical decisions. Theologians themselves will sometimes argue — and on the basis of convictions about God as Creator and Provider — that there are moral principles knowable by reason, but they need not pretend that such standards give a full or finally adequate account of the moral life. At any rate, more modest claims about the possibilities and promises of a common moral language may free religious persons and communities to rediscover their traditions, to recover their own voices, and to speak more eloquently in their own languages about medical ethics. More candidly theological talk about medicine and morals may at least remind a pluralistic culture of the minimal character of the standards it presumes are universal, rational, and sufficient.

Moreover, in spite of secularism, there are still many people who *are* believers. Indeed, more people who face choices about birth and death and suffering and about caring for those who suffer or die or give birth belong to religious communities than belong — as Gustafson and Hauerwas put it — to "that fictional denomination called rational moral agents to which our colleagues in moral philosophy seek to evangelize all of us" (Gustafson and Hauerwas 1979: 346). Members of religious communities — or many of them, at any rate — want to make these choices they face with religious integrity, not just with impartial rationality. For their sake especially — and not only for the sake of the field of medical ethics and the pluralistic society of which we are a part — it is important that the continuing tasks of rediscovering religious traditions and recovering religious voices be continually renewed.

A small part of that task of recovery and renewal is what is undertaken in this volume. As the theologians treated utilized their traditions faithfully and creatively, so their work becomes part of the tradition to be examined sympathetically but not uncritically. The authors of the essays in this book engage in some selective retrieval of the work of their teachers (whether or not they ever had their "teacher" for a class). They attempt again to rediscover a religious tradition and to recover a theological voice — to provide a remedy for the "discontents of secularism" or to serve the discourse and discernment of particular religious communities concerning medical ethics. And like Callahan's "short history," the essays included in this volume invite us toward a future in which religious traditions and theological voices will be restored to a prominent role in medical ethics. It is our hope that toward such a future these essays might point the way.

References

Callahan, Daniel. 1990. "Religion and the Secularization of Bioethics." *Hastings Center Report*, Special Supplement: "Theology, Religious Traditions, and Bioethics," 20, no. 4 (July/August): 2-4.

Gustafson, James M., and Stanley Hauerwas. 1979. "Editorial." *The Journal of Medicine and Philosophy* 4, no. 4 (December): 345-46.

Jakobovits, Immanuel. 1959. *Jewish Medical Ethics.* New York: Block.

MacIntyre, Alasdair. 1981. *After Virtue: A Study in Moral Theory.* Notre Dame: University of Notre Dame Press.

National Commission for the Protection of Human Subjects of Biomedical and Behavioral Research. 1978. *The Belmont Report.* Washington, D.C.: DHEW Publication No. (05) 78-0012.

Ramsey, Paul. 1970. *The Patient as Person: Explorations in Medical Ethics.* New Haven: Yale University Press.

Ramsey, Paul. 1974. "The Indignity of 'Death with Dignity.'" *Hastings Center Studies* 2, no. 2 (May): 47-62.

Stout, Jeffrey. 1988. *Ethics After Babel: The Language of Morals and Their Discontents.* Boston: Beacon Press.

Walters, LeRoy. 1985. "Religion and the Renaissance of Medical Ethics." In *Theology and Bioethics: Exploring the Foundation and Frontiers,* ed. Earl E. Shelp *(Philosophy and Medicine 20)*, 3-16. Dordrecht: D. Reidel Publishing Company.

ON PAUL RAMSEY

A Covenant-Centered Ethic for Medicine

DAVID H. SMITH

WITH THE publication of *The Patient as Person* in 1970, Paul Ramsey established himself as the most influential American Protestant writer on medical ethics of his generation. In the years following, Ramsey has always made it clear that he writes from a self-consciously theological perspective, although he has denied that this orientation limits the relevance of his normative conclusions. Unfortunately, however, Ramsey's conclusions are often better known than his rationale for them, a situation exacerbated by the difficulty of his prose. In these pages I offer a short synopsis of Ramsey's general theological perspective and then show how it affects his analysis of issues in medical ethics. Since my personal and intellectual debts to Ramsey are large, I cannot claim detachment, but I may be able to offer a critical reading that opens the insights and limits of Ramsey's perspective to further scrutiny.[1]

I

The first step in understanding Paul Ramsey's moral theory is to recognize that it is controlled and informed by prior faith commitments:

---

1. For some other discussions of Ramsey's work, see Curran 1973; Cahill 1975; and Johnson and Smith 1974. Ramsey's response to the last can be found in Ramsey 1976.

it is covenant-centered. Its basis is the assumption that God has made a covenant with people and that people therefore have an obligation to be faithful to that covenant. This assumption has two components. The first is God's establishment of a bond with humankind. So far as I know, Ramsey has never tried to *prove* that this bond exists — although he would not admit that belief in its existence is irrational. The second ingredient we might call a principle of replication. As God has committed himself to us, so ought we to commit ourselves to each other. The God-human relationship establishes a standard or norm for person-to-person relationships. This fundamental starting point clearly has much in common with the thought of such neoorthodox theologians as Anders Nygren, Karl Barth, and H. Richard Niebuhr.

Ramsey develops these foundational ideas most thoroughly in *Basic Christian Ethics* (1950), in which he argues that fidelity to the action of God requires congruent fidelity between persons. Therefore "Christian ethics is a deontological ethics," and "neighbor love is not good, it is obligatory" (1950: 115, 116). Right relations, faithful relations between persons are all-important: "The Christian understanding of righteousness is . . . radically non-teleological. It means ready obedience to the *present* reign of God, the alignment of the human will with the Divine will that men should live together in covenant-love no matter what the morrow brings, even if it brings nothing" (1967: 108).

It is characteristic that Ramsey explains the requirements of covenant-love in terms of need. "The biblical notion of justice," he writes, "may be summed up in the principle: To each according to the measure of his real need, not because of anything human reason can discern inherent in the needy, but because his need alone is the measure of God's righteousness towards him" (1950: 14). He presents this as the core of the Old Testament teaching, but he finds the basic idea continued in the New Testament. Early Christians regarded Jesus as the center of the covenant; he embodied and taught the importance of love (1950: 14-24). The love commandment is the basic rule or principle of Christian ethics. "Everything is lawful, *absolutely everything* is permitted which love permits, everything without a single exception." And "*absolutely everything* is commanded which love requires, absolutely everything without the slightest exception or softening" (1950: 89).

Ramsey's view of the relationship between eschatology, or beliefs about ultimate destiny, and ethics in the teachings of Jesus has given his stress on the needs of a neighbor a characteristic twist. He maintains that Jesus' teaching was apocalyptic, that is, that Jesus expected the world to be radically transformed — and soon. For Ramsey, that means that it was directed to the relationship between only two individuals. Jesus was primarily concerned with the proper form of that relationship.

Ramsey's argument is ingenious. Jesus, he claims, expected an immediate transformation of the world by God. This transformation would establish a historical reign of absolute justice. Thus when Jesus commanded his followers to love, he did not expect love "to be able to deal with every form of evil"; he assigned to it a "limited but positively creative function" (1950: 37-39). Jesus' eschatology limited the sphere of his ethical concern. Does this limitation invalidate the ethic in an age that does not share the literal hopes of the teacher? No, because we can mentally strip away concern for the future as Jesus' beliefs forced him to do. For us the eschatological situation, the morally decisive fact, is the relation with one particular other person. Jesus' commandment to love provides us with a norm for that one relationship. It shows me how I ought to be related to each of the many other persons with whom I come in contact.

Thus the apocalyptic element, which appeared to be a liability in the teaching of Jesus, turns out to be its strongest asset. Of course we live in a world of many personal relationships, but social conditions and problems change, and a generally relevant, policy oriented ethic becomes dated. To achieve eternal relevance, "we need to see clearly how we should be obliged to behave toward one neighbor . . . if there were no other claims on us at all" (1950: 44). Very briefly:

> Christian ethics may claim to be relevant in criticism of every situation precisely because its standard . . . is not accommodated to man's continuing life in normal historical relationships; and this in turn is true in point of origin precisely because of Jesus' apocalyptic view of the kingdom of God. (1950: 44; cf. 42)

There is real continuity between the Christian and Jesus. Jesus demanded total concern for the needs of each neighbor. The Christian can abstract himself or herself from an actual plurality of relationships and use the standard of the love commandment to measure each relationship.

Ramsey (1962) has subsequently modified his view of New Testament eschatology, but his ethical analyses are best seen as rooted in the intellectual maneuver just described. The modification has allowed Ramsey to put behind him the manifold and complicated text of the New Testament: for him the New Testament ethic is the demand of faithful love between neighbors. But distilling the New Testament ethic to the command to serve the needs of a neighbor creates a new set of problems.

The first problems cluster around the question, Which neighbor? From the very first, Ramsey has produced two answers. Sometimes he adopts what can only be described as a positivistic answer: The neighbor to be served is the one you find yourself related to and are able to serve. Thus, for instance, Christian love means an entirely "neighbor-regarding concern for others which begins with the first man it sees" (1950: 95). On the other hand, Ramsey sometimes uses a "degrees of need" test, in which one is most obliged to the neediest individual. Thus in *Basic Christian Ethics* he argues for a "redemptive" definition of justice "with special bias in favor of the helpless who can contribute nothing at all and are in fact 'due' nothing" (1950: 14). On the whole I think it fair to say that Ramsey means to begin with the first criterion and then apply the second. That is, the field of responsibilities is primarily restricted by de facto relationships and then, within this field, one is biased toward the most needy.

The problem becomes more acute when we realize that people face not only alternative but *competing* claims. Not only may the needs of any two individuals be so great as to demand more than we can give; beyond that, their needs may conflict. Jesus did not feel he had to adjudicate conflicting claims, but the Christian must take responsibility for such judgments (1967: 33). Of course the problem becomes especially difficult in medicine, when life and death are at stake.

The clearest example of Ramsey's discussion of this issue in the medical sphere concerns the allocation of scarce medical resources. He notices that there will never be enough time, pharmacology, technology, or donated tissue to meet all human need. Some can be saved, but not all. What does Christianity require in this situation? Ramsey rejects any sort of value-laden choices among individuals. Rather, he argues, the only legitimate basis for choice among patients is random selection, or its closest social equivalent, a first-come, first-served system. The obvious inequalities among persons are irrelevant "in deciding who lives and who dies." And they are irrelevant because all lives are of equal worth in the sight of God. In a lottery or first-come, first-served system human beings "stand aside as far as possible from the choice of who shall live and who shall die" (1970a: 255, 256). Ramsey is critical of policies that reward or encourage sensational treatments for a few as opposed to mundane help for many (1970a: 268). But the interesting theoretical point is the extent to which his understanding of the Christian ethic controls the kind of issue he finds it appropriate to try to adjudicate. Far from providing a criterion for deciding who should receive care, Christian love says, in effect, this issue is outside my scope. Triage, choosing those most needed, is plausible only in a small community whose *survival* is clearly dependent on given individuals (1970a: 258, 275).

Another way to look at the issue of resource allocation is to see it as an issue of *what* is needed; several kinds of needs should have priority. Is it more important to find a cure for cancer, develop an artificial heart, or work on cures for arthritis? What is the relative importance of preventive and therapeutic medicine? Indeed, what is the relative importance of health care, education, and defense?

Ramsey is unwilling on principle to pronounce on these kinds of questions. He opts for social discussion of the issue, rather than pontification by the moralist (1970a: 275). This deference is rooted first in Ramsey's view that the question of *what* is needed is a secondary issue: "When right relation to neighbor has been established, then and only then does Christian love need to become as enlightened as possible about what is truly good for the neighbor" (1950: 116; cf. 142). But what is secondary is not unimportant.

This deference is also rooted in Ramsey's view that a moralist's own perceptions of what is valuable or shoddy must not be canonized. He resists writing in ways that suggest that he is himself an unusually discerning or sensitive perceiver of what is good or bad in the world. To enter into those kinds of judgments would seem to him presumptuous. The moralist, he has said, is an expert on duties or "canons of loyalty," not on material descriptions of what people need. His postulates about need really boil down to needs for consensual community and for protection.

With *Nine Modern Moralists*, Ramsey begins using individual case histories to support the notion that we have a "sense of injustice" (1962: chaps. 8, 9). He argues that love "begins with persons and then devolves or discerns the rules. . . . The Christian starts with people and not rules

11

... with the multiple claims and needs of his neighbors" (1967: 111).[2] Principles are products of the *relationship* between lover and neighbor. Once need has been discerned in a case, love or *agape* adds an ingredient of fidelity, loyalty, or constancy. If a neighbor needs X, then *agape* unequivocally requires that a Christian provide it.

In this context we can see the senses in which Ramsey is, and is not, a "situationalist." Insofar as situationism means a willingness to reformulate, he has no quarrel with it. New problems and cases should force the Christian "to specify as aptly as possible the meaning of faithfulness to other men required by the particular covenants or causes between us" (Ramsey 1968a: 125). The root problem of situationism is not unwillingness to generalize but inability to see that absolute commitment to the neighbor *means* exceptionless (that is, constant) commitment to his or her need. On Ramsey's terms, to surrender constant commitment to the neighbor's need would be to surrender the Christian ethic. Of course we must reformulate, but our added experience will "only disclose deeper meanings as to how faithfulness within relations should shape our behavior" (Ramsey 1968a: 127).

Another important theme in Ramsey's formulation of Christian ethics is the idea that the world is God's creation, dependent on God for its being, order, and future. Ramsey makes use of this notion as a way of establishing the equal worth of all people, whatever their social status. It also lies behind his case method of discerning need, for the theological premise of that method is the idea that crucial determinants of what the Christian should do emerge from study of the historical world, rather than from revelation.

To date Ramsey has not developed the methodological structure for use of the creation theme in nearly the detail with which he has refined the covenant theme. But it is associated with some distinctive features of his thought. For example, Ramsey has a most sympathetic reading of pre–Vatican II Catholic moral theology and of casuistry generally. The willingness of the Catholic casuists — and of Aquinas and Augustine — to look at cases certainly suits Ramsey's temperament and instructs him. But the root of this sympathy is the shared conviction

2. On the difficult topic of Ramsey and "exceptionless moral rules," see the excellent article by Donald Evans, "Paul Ramsey on Exceptionless Moral Rules," in Johnson and Smith 1974: 19-46, and Ramsey's reply in "Some Rejoinders" (1976).

that God reigns over all and that we can discern something of the normative structure of the creation.

Second, Ramsey clearly interprets this total dependence upon God to imply the equal sanctity of all human life. This postulate is central in his discussions of the definition of death, abortion, and genetic engineering. A fundamental issue in those arguments, of course, concerns what one means by a human relation to God, upon whom we confess our dependence. The covenant-affirming side of Ramsey's intellectual persona could read this relationship as a *conscious* relation to God. The implication would be that human beings lacking such a relation were subpersonal, not in God's image, and therefore of diminished importance. An exclusive stress on covenant could cohere with a neocortical definition of death — one that makes the possibility of consciousness central — and a low view of the status of human embryos and fetuses. The fact that Ramsey finds these conclusions abhorrent reflects his deep commitment to a supplementary theme of creation, the idea that the central root of human value lies in the relation to a creator, a relation not dependent upon human capacity for awareness. God's creation need not be *aware* of God in the same sense that God's covenant partner must.

Obviously the creation postulate qualifies the covenant theme in a conservative direction, and another complication in Ramsey's thought confirms this direction. Ramsey has a very strong sense of the brokenness of the world as we know it. He has seen suffering firsthand; hopes for a world without conflict, disappointment, death, and suffering always strike him as unrealistic. This realism is evident in his discussion of resource allocation, and it comes up again and again in his work on medical ethics.

II

Before we turn our attention to medical ethics, it will be helpful to illustrate Ramsey's way of reasoning with reference to a general problem. Are Christians ever able to justify killing? Prohibitions on lying and on killing have been important parts of the Christian ethical tradition. Although Ramsey has not written much about the former issue, the latter has been a major, perhaps the central, subject of his work for over forty years. Obviously his starting point must be a commitment to the needs of another. Can this commitment justify taking a life? Ramsey's answer is yes — if the killing is necessary in order to protect another, innocent person. If the only parties to a conflict situation are the Christian and someone who threatens him or her, then the Christian is obliged to die rather than kill. But this is virtually never the case. More than one relationship must always be considered. We have to face the question of love for the threatened other.

Jesus' apocalyptic or eschatological ethic was pacifistic. It referred directly to the one-to-one relationship. Our forms of responsibility are more complicated, so we must ask about the implications of full fidelity, if a *third party's* life is threatened.

> Jesus dealt only with the simplest moral situation in which blows may be struck, the case of one person in relation to but one other. He does not .. undertake to say how men . . . ought to act in more complex cases where non-resistance would in practice mean turning another person's face to the blows of an oppressor. (1950: 167)

My love for one neighbor may require me to be violent to another one. I am to love person X; X is attacked by person Y; out of love for X, I am required to do violence to Y. My prior commitment to someone in need of protection is more important than a general abstract rule.

Notice that for Ramsey Christian love doesn't just tolerate killing to protect — it requires it. He rejects the idea that this situation is too awful for love to be relevant. The irrelevance of love to any human decision is the one thing that Ramsey will never concede. Rather than implying the irrelevance of love, a tragic situation puts love to the test. The depth of my commitment to the neighbor is, in a way, revealed in what I am willing to do for him or her. What kind of *agape* can I be said to have for X if I refuse to protect X from harm? "Participation in regrettable conflict falls among distasteful tasks which sometimes become imperative for Christian vocation. Only one thing is necessary: for love's sake it must be done" (1950: 184). The justification of such behavior has nothing to do with the "superiority" of the Christian; it has everything to do with the moral trump: the concrete need of a particular neighbor for protection (1950: 179). The crucial Christian principle is the duty to protect the weak.

III

With this background let us turn to some specific topics in medical ethics. Abortion is the first issue related to medicine that Ramsey wrote about. Particularly important for him is the question of fetal humanity (see Ramsey 1968b). Most of his discussions of abortion presuppose the human status of the fetus, and I will take up that topic in the next section. A second crucial aspect of this issue concerns loyalty to fetuses. May they ever be killed? Ramsey's view on this issue has remained quite constant: fetuses may be killed only in order to protect life. That is, Ramsey applies the paradigm I discussed above, seeing the fetus as the innocent and threatened party.

Interestingly, his first discussion of abortion occurs in *War and the Christian Conscience* (1961). Ramsey describes the traditional Roman Catholic position on abortion, which holds that direct (that is, intentional and immediate) killing is always wrong. Thus surgery that directly kills a fetus is prohibited. If fetal life and maternal life conflict, and if the only way to save the mother is by directly killing the fetus, then nothing may be done. It is better to let both die than to kill directly.

The substance of Ramsey's disagreement with this position has never changed, but his language has. In earlier writings he maintains that the problem with the Catholic alternative is that it fails "to allow charity any vital role in the matter of morality" (1961: 176).

> By the absolutely supreme end of *agape,* not every means, not even every indispensable means, is justified, but surely every means to save life the only alternative to which is . . . death. . . . To make this choice, on behalf of life and against death and inaction, is not to do wrong but to do what we know to be right. (1961: 186)

Ramsey repeats his basic paradigm in which fidelity to one person can justify killing, and he goes on to say that the observable "directness" of the killing does not count against the basic obligations involved.

In Ramsey's subsequent discussions of abortion even these killings are not intentional. Thus, in "The Morality of Abortion" (1968b), he argues that direct abortions are justified in situations where a nonviable fetus threatens its mother's life. In that case:

> the intention of the action, and *in this sense its direction,* is not upon

15

the *death* of the foetus . . . [but it is] directed toward the *incapacitation* of the foetus from doing what it is doing to the life of the mother. (1968b: 84; first italics added)

The intention of the action is not fetal death but "incapacitation." The crucial fact is "the child's functional relation to its mother's death" (1973: 174-226), which produces a situation in which

an *observable, physically direct killing* of an unborn child should be understood to have the intention of *stopping* its lethal action upon its mother's life and not to have the objective of killing that child as such apart from its fatal function. (1973: 220)

This distinction between incapacitation and direct killing solves the problem of explaining how love can justify abortion. If justifiable abortions are properly described as incapacitating rather than killing, then one can say that such actions are justifiable as acts of love to the aborted fetus. One has not done something unloving to the fetus in itself. The question is whether the distinction between incapacitation and killing can be sustained. The difference cannot be explained in terms of effects on the fetus or a description of medical movements leading to its death. In an individualistic focus on the death of one being, both an "incapacitating" and a wicked action of life taking are killing.

The key to the distinction is the concept of intention. Intention, as we ordinarily use the word, as Thomas Aquinas seemed to use it, and as Ramsey uses it, has a decisively contextual referent. It is not simply a description of an event in abstraction from the relations among the parties. Properly understood, intention must be seen as part of a narrative.

In Ramsey's writing on abortion we can test the intention in an act of killing by asking whether we would kill the individual if we were not in this particular situation. The important issue is "whether we would save the child's life if we could, if it were not inexorably bringing about the death of his mother (and his own) or fatally in the way of [that is, obstructing] actions to save her" (1973: 222; cf. 221). Given the fetus's biological role, surgically killing it is better described as justified abortion than direct feticide. Roles and relationships thus are decisive for the significance of action (1968b: 85); judgments about the final worth of persons, about their relation to God, vastly exceed our power.

The test of this analysis occurs when the only way to make a decision seems to be comparative worth, when there is mutual threat and one partner, but not both, can survive. If one must choose between mother and fetus, then Ramsey's initial instinct was that we should "randomize" the choice (1973: 220 n. 25). Because human sovereignty is limited, it is never acceptable to fall back on comparative worth; justification for protection must be found in the possibility of protecting one party from the threat of another. But his final judgment is that a third party (for example, the husband) could choose for the mother because of her obligations to the children or himself (1976: 193).

Ramsey's subsequent writings on abortion reflect these same concerns. Although he will allow the logical possibility that socioeconomic factors may mean that pregnancy poses a threat to maternal life, for example, for a poor woman living on the margin, he is skeptical of the general validity of this argument (1971: 17). Generally, he has been dismayed at the course of American abortion law and practice since *Roe v. Wade,* the 1973 Supreme Court decision that states may not ban abortions. Thus he has insisted that effects on the fetus do make some techniques for abortion preferable over others and that live abortuses should be accorded equal status with infants birthed normally (1970: chap. 1). He thinks it is mistaken to relate the issue of fetal sanctity to the question of fetal location by suggesting that the fetus has lower status in utero (1978: 110-12).

It is inevitable that these claims will be provocative to some feminists, but Ramsey's main target is individualism. Simply to say to women "you are responsible for your own decisions and their consequences" is to him an act of betrayal. In fact, Ramsey's work over the past ten years reflects a strong preoccupation with community and (as Gilbert Meilaender pointed out to me) with *law*. He is troubled by solitary decision making about abortion (1978: chap. 1). And he thinks there must be collective, institutional support for physicians and nurses whose consciences cannot tolerate a liberal policy. Somehow the law must be changed, for more than maternal rights is at stake (1978: 115). "In matters so basic as slavery and the taking of life, one who believes either to be wrong cannot fail to advocate public and legal policy prohibiting such action" (1978: 87 n. 38). He considers a moderate law that would allow abortions after viability only for the sake of maternal health. Would it be constitutional? To be morally credible a strict definition of threat to health would be necessary; viability would have to be defined conservatively (if any doubt, a ruling of viable), and that definition would be subject to regular updating.

I am persuaded that Ramsey's treatment of abortion is controlled by his concern for protection — not only of fetuses but of women. If he is mistaken, the root cause may be an overly strong sense of women's need for protection; in any event one could modify his *policy* recommendations greatly by developing a democratic argument to the effect that within certain limits abortion decisions appropriately devolve on pregnant women.

IV

Ramsey's treatment of the abortion issue encapsulates most of the main themes in his other writing in the field of medical ethics. Abortion obviously raises questions about who counts as a member of the human community. Ramsey's conviction is that all human beings have a special kind of sanctity because all are God's children. If we doubt whether a given individual belongs in the human community, Ramsey's principle is to be inclusive.

Thus, in considering the moral status of fetuses, Ramsey discusses two extreme options. In one option humanity is associated with the capacity for personal interaction. But personal interaction is a vague term, and its use as a criterion can have the effect of excluding children and others who, it seems obvious to Ramsey, must count as human beings. The alternative Ramsey calls a genetic theory: roughly, that whenever the human chromosome count is present in an organism, then that organism is a human being of the same status as the rest of us. Ramsey comes close to accepting this view. Part of his reason for rejecting it concerns identical twins who might, on the genetic theory, be said to have only one identity. Thus Ramsey suggests that characteristically human status should be said to begin when an individuated member of the human species exists — at the blastocyst stage, with segmentation or twinning (1971: 5 n. 1).

He goes on to argue that this debate is not very important after all, because, he insists, the basis for human sanctity is not a human property but God's graciousness:

> The value of a human life is ultimately grounded in the value God is placing on it. . . . [M]an is a sacredness in human biological processes

no less than he is a sacredness in the human social or political order. That sacredness is not composed by observable degrees of relative worth. A life's sanctity consists not in its worth to anybody. What life is in and of itself is most clearly to be seen in situations of naked equality of one life with another, and in the situation of congeneric helplessness which is the human condition in the first of life. No one is ever much more than a fellow fetus. . . . (1971: 12)

What Ramsey means to reject is clear enough. But an issue remains, and we can get at it if we make a distinction between the source of human sanctity and the *presence* or *manifestation* of that sanctity. Presumably God is the source of the sanctity of the entire creation — God is related not only to human beings. Ramsey will never deny God's omnipotence. But then the question becomes, How can we differentiate God's special relationship to human beings from his relationship to the rest of the created order? What evidence might we give to show that a given being is of the kind that the special sanctity is present with it or manifest toward it? Thoughtful Christian and Jewish persons disagree over the question of whether early fetuses fall within the special sanctity penumbra, and it is of no help in argumentation to remind them that the *source* of dignity is God.

Ramsey rightly sees this point, and he takes a position on when human dignity begins. The possible mistake lies in his suggestion that the issue of a starting point may not be important in theological morality. In general, Ramsey's position on fetal sanctity fits much better with his stress on creation than it does with the more dominant emphasis on covenant in his work. He comes close to affirming that the image of God is bodily and denies that the essentially human is simply the socially relational.

We see some of these same emphases in Ramsey's discussion of the definition of death. Here he insists that we distinguish the *concept* of death from the *criteria* used in determining whether someone has died. Ramsey means to allow medical science great latitude on the question of criteria and favors use of something like the "Harvard Report" tests of absence of reflexes, responses, and respiration, but he insists that the concept of death should not be altered so that humans who are permanently comatose are counted as dead. As with fetuses, inability to relate humanly is not sufficient evidence that special human dignity has been lost. When in doubt, opt for inclusion.

19

It is quite characteristic of Ramsey to refuse to conflate the questions of status and care. That is, he insists that we first debate the status issue and then discuss what loyalty to the patient may require. Shortcuts are possible. It is tempting, as a practical matter, to say, "Well, whatever it (patient or fetus) is, it certainly doesn't matter much. No harm is done by shortening its life, and others may be greatly assisted." Ramsey sets his face against this rationalization with the tenacity of the best of his Protestant forebears. For the conflation leads inevitably to a devaluing of the life that cannot speak for itself. It is possible that more refined neurological criteria can be formulated, and Ramsey has no problem with the use of neurological criteria per se. But until we have absolutely reliable tests for central nervous system activity, "deeply comatose patients, the tragic 'vegetable' cases whose respiration and hearts continue naturally, fall under an ethics of caring for the dying, the not yet dead, perhaps even the not yet dying" (1970a: 90 n. 37).

V

Ramsey also discusses in his writings on medical ethics the ways in which reproduction might be controlled. He begins by noting that his work depends on a characteristically Christian interpretation of the world, one in which God's sovereignty over the creation is central. A more secular eschatology stakes everything on the fate of humankind. Unfortunate genetic outcomes — whether for individuals or species — are ultimate evils. In contrast, Christian eschatology suggests that human existence is meaningless apart from God's providence and that we must focus our attention upon the *means* for attaining good ends.

> [A]ny person, or any society or age, expecting ultimate success where ultimate success is not to be reached, is peculiarly apt to devise extreme and morally illegitimate means for getting there. . . . [M]en have another end than the receding future contains. (1970b: 31)

Not only is ultimate preoccupation with outcomes likely to be morally mischievous, our goals may change. One epoch's values are not those of another (1970b: 56). Affirmation of God's rule means accepting the parameters of human existence (for example, its generational structure). Radically recreating humankind amounts to a kind of "species

20

suicide" and the upshot is "man's limitless dominion over man" (1970b: 152).

Ramsey is open to a variety of means to try to ameliorate the human prospect, but he does rule out altogether two kinds of intentionality. The first concerns separating acts of reproduction from acts of love. Ramsey's argument on this point is imaginative and difficult.

He begins with the observation that Christians confess the singularity of God's relationship with the world. For example, it is easy to imagine a mythology in which God loves one world and creates another. But that is not the biblical imagery; there God has a complex relationship of creation and covenant — with one and the same "partner" world.

> God created nothing apart from His love; and without the divine love was not anything made that was made. Neither should there be among men and women . . . any love set out of the context of responsibility for procreation, any begetting apart from the sphere of love. A reflection of God's love . . . is found in the claim He placed upon men and women in their creation when He bound the nurturing of marital love and procreation together in the nature of human sexuality. (1970b: 38)

Ramsey uses here the same principle of replication that is foundational in his ethics: Christian bonds of loyalty are to replicate the archetypal bond established by God. People should not separate procreative from loving acts on principle. On the one hand, this means no adultery; on the other, it means no use of donated gametes: no artificial insemination by donor and no egg donors. It does not preclude contraception, for that does not separate the essential components of the relationship.

In fact, the love-procreation link does not require reproduction at all. Ramsey is clear that genetic reasons may be appropriate for the vocation of childlessness (1970b: 38); indeed, he insists that a couple has no right to have a child (1970b: 120). His point is that use of surrogate mothers or gamete donors violates something that is essential to humankind as we understand it to be: a yoking of loving and begetting.

But we can exploit other parties besides each other. Chief among them is the new life we may beget. This young life comes into the world at some risk, and the irony is that the only way we can test the risk is by subjecting some young humans to it. On the one hand is the raw risk, the chance that the child may be born impaired or that its parents may reject it. But the more serious issue is the damage to the child's moral status: it has been asked to run a risk when, in the nature of the case, it could not possibly have consented. The full force of this claim will emerge in the discussion of Ramsey's views on experimentation.

Ramsey's willingness to follow the logical implications of these views illustrates the subtlety of his mind as well as the perseverance of his disposition.[3] Unfortunately some of the argumentation is accessible to only the most dedicated of Ramsey's readers.

VI

The concerns of Ramsey's discussed so far have been substantive rather than procedural — concerns about what we should do rather than about who should decide. But his contribution on the latter topic has been enormous, particularly in his treatment of the morality of experimentation.

Ramsey begins with the assumption that the relationship between subject and researcher must be a relationship between persons. That is, both roles of the relationship count. Thus, for Ramsey, the first question to be asked is, What are the morally relevant features of the relationship between researcher and subject?

Ramsey suggests in effect that the research relationship should be *contrasted* with the therapeutic relationship. Even the nomenclature is different. In the therapeutic context we speak of a physician (or other healer) and a patient; in the research context we refer to an investigator and a subject. The reason for this difference in terms has to do with the purpose of the procedure. The objective of therapy is the benefit of the patient, but the purpose of experimentation is benefit for someone *other than* the patient.

Ramsey's reflections on experimentation all work with this rather narrow definition of what constitutes an experiment. His primary concern is not the existence or degree of *risk*. Rather, for him, the essence of an experiment is the fact that it is not meant to benefit the person on whom procedures, pharmacology, or devices are tested.

3. See, among others, his essay "The Issues Facing Mankind," in Lejeune, Ramsey, and Wright 1984: 19-46.

Ramsey contends that consent is necessary for both therapy and experimental procedures. His argument is twofold. On the one hand, humans as conscious subjects have the capacity to agree to let others touch and influence their bodies; on the other hand, because we are likely to abuse our power, it is important that our jurisdiction over each other be limited by the agreement of the weaker party. These points are especially important in the case of experimentation. Ramsey adapts Reinhold Niebuhr's statement that "man's capacity for justice makes democracy possible; man's capacity for injustice makes democracy necessary." As adapted the argument reads: "Man's capacity to become joint adventurers in a common cause makes the consensual relation possible; man's propensity to overreach his joint adventurer even in a good cause makes consent necessary" (1970a: 5). People have the right to use their bodies for the benefit of humankind, if they choose to do so. That is the positive argument for experimentation as a human endeavor rooted in consent. But people also have a tendency to abuse the persons over whom they have power. That is the negative warrant for consent: to keep researchers from exploiting subjects.

In the case of therapy we allow proxy consent; we say that it is acceptable for one person to consent on someone else's behalf. It would be foolish to prohibit treatment on someone, perhaps lifesaving treatment, because that person had not consented. Most of us would object if emergency lifesaving treatment were withheld from us because we had not consented. And it is that intuition that lies behind the widespread acceptance of proxy consent for therapy.

But benefit of the person touched is exactly what we cannot assume in the case of experimentation. Therefore to allow proxy consent for experimentation is morally unjustifiable. Proxy consent for risky therapy is another matter. As long as there is plausible hope that the procedure or therapy will benefit the person touched — that is, as long as it is accurate to describe this person as a patient rather than a subject — Ramsey has no problem with proxy consent. However, in experimental procedures, designed to benefit others, there is no plausible rationale for proxy consent. Ramsey's core principle is simple: no experimentation without consent.

Ramsey follows this principle with relentless consistency. If a subject cannot consent, then he or she cannot legitimately be a subject. Thus: no experimentation on children or the comatose, even if the risks to them are very small. The issue for Ramsey is not risk; it is consent.

If something is done to me that I do not agree to, I am exploited, I am insulted as a person, even if I am not harmed. Uninjured, I remain insulted.

Rejecting strong forms of the argument that institutionalization makes consent impossible, Ramsey denies that experiments on prisoners are intrinsically immoral. But he would discourage them because of the inherently coercive character of institutional life. And research on institutionalized children is not just morally wrong but, on Ramsey's terms, should be outlawed.

The discussion of experimentation that Ramsey engaged in for about ten years beautifully illustrates certain aspects of his thought. One is its rigorism. On Ramsey's terms Christian love must mean protecting possible subjects from exploitation. Standing for that protection is an exceptionless rule — or nearly so. Yet it is not clear exactly how large is the class of cases to which this rule applies, for almost all clinical experimentation seems to have a possible benefit for the patient and it is thus, on Ramsey's terms, not really *experimentation* but *risky therapy*. In a sense Ramsey may be too tolerant of abuses associated with therapeutic clinical research.

Second, it illustrates the Ramsey's relationalism. The insight that gets his whole analysis off the ground is, in effect, a kind of phenomenological distinction between two seemingly similar but essentially different forms of human relationship. His general point is that some kinds of action are inconsistent with a certain kind of relation.

But finally it illustrates the concern for physical protection of weak individuals that is part of Ramsey's thought, a fact that has clearly come out in his discussions about this subject with Richard McCormick, S.J. McCormick's more Catholic vision allows for the possibility that low-risk nontherapeutic experiments on children might be justified in a few cases. For Ramsey this sanctifying possibility must be a matter of individual choice. His stress on protecting the individual from abuse necessarily deemphasizes the extent to which the individual can receive support from the community.

VII

Ramsey's first major discussion of the care of the dying occurs in *The Patient as Person* (1970a), and in my judgment the third chapter of that book remains one of Ramsey's most significant pieces of work. Ramsey's thought on caring for the dying is relational through and through. Individuals differ, so the demands of care for one individual are different from those of care for another. Yet all individuals die, and their proper care will take that fact into account. Appropriate norms are a function of the objectively changing situation of the patient for whom others care.

Before a patient begins to die, loyalty to that patient, or care, requires skilled work to cure his or her diseases. But once the patient starts to die, the requirements of care enter a new phase. It no longer makes sense to say that the patient needs *cure*. Now the most serious problems are discomfort and loneliness. Medical care for the dying instead requires providing *comfort*, that is, symptom control and company.

For Ramsey, it is a mistake to focus on a distinction between omission and commission. If a patient is dying, then a decision not to give an injection or start a respirator is not an omission but a recognition that needs have changed. It is most accurate to describe this action as "ceasing to do something that was begun in order to do something that is better because now more fitting" (1970a: 151; cf. 144-53, 132-36). Actions of technologically limited but humanly appropriate care for the dying are totally different from positive euthanasia, which on Ramsey's terms represents the crucial moral omission, namely, omission to care for the dying as long as it is humanly possible.

Ramsey concludes his first discussion of care for the dying by specifying circumstances in which mercy killing might be permissible. The two classes of cases he contemplates are deeply comatose patients and those whose pain cannot be assuaged. Should either of these conditions proceed to the point at which "it is entirely indifferent to the patient" whether death comes sooner or later, then and only then might direct killing be considered. If the patient can no longer be ministered to by another person, then the issue of care is taken out of human hands (1970a: 160-64). If we can no longer meet the needs of living persons (and these patients certainly are alive on Ramsey's terms), then the rationale for our obligations to them can no longer be developed in the covenantal context.

Notice that the linchpin of this discussion is a judgment about the beginning of the dying process, which only a physician can make (1970a: 132-36). But it is not entirely clear what the physician is looking for. We could clear up the obscurities in either of two ways. The decisive point might be understood to be (1) the time when the patient (or a proxy) decides that continued life is undesirable; or (2) a time after which life is no longer worth living — when the patient's quality of life is so low that it seems cruel to continue to treat him or her. Either of these ways of understanding the time at which the requirements of care change would be politically clearer than the criterion Ramsey was looking for, but anyone who has followed thus far will anticipate that Ramsey cannot possibly accept them.

From Ramsey's point of view, making the patient's choice the decisive criterion "enthrones . . . an arbitrary freedom," or, put differently, "there are medically indicated treatments . . . that a competent conscious patient has no moral right to refuse, just as *no one has a moral right deliberately to ruin his health*." Rather than stressing the patient's absolute right to refuse treatment, we should "emphasize his free and informed *participation* in medical decisions affecting him when there are alternative treatments" (1978: 156-57; italics added).

Ramsey rejects the second option, focusing on the quality of the patient's life, on several grounds. He resists the idea that an end of human achievement, in particular the impossibility for a relationship with another human, represents a signal from God that it is time for the patient to die. Moreover, he does not see how social and psychological factors can be excluded from the factors that influence quality of life. Socioeconomic factors also can give us good reason to predict a low quality of life. "Defenses of the benign neglect of defective newborns are also arguments for the benign neglect of at least some of the environmentally deprived" (1978: 176). So long as the patient is a person valued by God, we must ask about claims on us for our care (1978: 178). How can there be a life we *can* help that we do not have a *duty* to help? A need we *can* meet that we do not have a *duty* to meet?

Ramsey's rejection of these alternatives rests firmly on his most fundamental principles. Loyalty to the weak cannot be canceled simply because the weak become weaker. And the core moral principle is not individual self-determination but service to needy others. An ethic of care for the dying that takes as its central principle the right to refuse treatment — even if the decisive refusals must be reasonable — is simply operating in a different moral universe from the one Ramsey presupposes. If I identify myself with the ill patient, the problem with the stress on individual rights is that I exaggerate my own sovereignty over myself; if I identify myself with the caregiver, the problem with more voluntarist theories is loss of focus on the demand to do what I can. Both the stress on self-determination and that on quality of life ignore the covenantal principle of replication and the sovereignty of the creator.

Thus Ramsey falls back on a "medical indications" policy in which attention focuses on the condition of the patient rather than on any human being's choices or opinions about what makes life worth living (1978: 159). A competent adult has a "relative" right to refuse treatment. If the patient is unconscious but not dying, the only morally legitimate options are forms of care that not only provide comfort but preserve life whenever possible, except in cases where care doesn't reach. If, in contrast to these situations, the patient is dying, then it is legitimate to choose between treatments that will extend life and those — perhaps less onerous — that will not (1978: 165).

Obviously this conclusion can be described as paternalistic,[4] but the hard question is whether a more liberty-centered option is theologically credible. The alternatives of comparing the quality of lives and suggesting that some are "not worth living" or asserting that anything persons choose to do with themselves is ipso facto to be accepted are hard to reconcile with covenant bonding to a sovereign creator. Of course, a theological ethic can be centered on the theme of God's liberating salvation, but that would be a very different ethic from Ramsey's and would likely have significant omissions of its own. Perhaps it is no small compliment to say of Ramsey that he puts the ambiguity, the uncertainty, in the right place.

Ramsey applies these principles to several highly controversial situations. One of them is the problem of proper forms of care for handicapped newborns. Ramsey insists that to be born defective is not the same thing as to be born dying. Even a child with Tay-Sachs disease (a metabolic disorder that causes death usually before age three) is not dying yet; affliction with the pathology that will lead to death is not the same thing as dying (1978: 187, 191). "The standard for letting die must be the same for the normal child as for the defective child" (1978: 154). Refusal to treat is justified only if "there is special medical reason for saying the treatment might make them worse and in any case would

---

4. For a powerful example of this criticism of Ramsey's "medical indications" policy, see Childress 1982: 164ff.

not help. The comparison should be between treatments measured to the need" of the particular patient (1978: 194). Some babies may be beyond the reach of care — but not many. Certainly not infants with Down's syndrome.

*   *   *

Paul Ramsey's work in medical ethics has deep theological roots and is in many ways controlled by his theological vision of the world. For instance, it is that theological perspective which prevents him from building his discussion of care for the dying around the principle of the right to refuse treatment. Moreover, his theological perspective includes components — in particular the concept of loyalty — that have remarkably deep resonances in the common conscience. Indeed, Ramsey's vision of the life of covenant fidelity remains one of the most morally compelling to have been produced in this century.

Within that vision some of the most difficult issues concern the concept of need. A stronger commitment to autonomy, to a need for self-respect, would mean that respecting the right of self-determination is of a different order than meeting other needs. And Ramsey could, on principle, allow that a patient has a "need to die" — a need that is frustrated by a perverse medical technology. The fact that Ramsey does not draw these conclusions reflects his remarkable lifelong preoccupation with the protection of the weak. If that is a mistake, it is easy to imagine worse ones.

References

Cahill, Lisa S. 1975. "Paul Ramsey: Covenant Fidelity in Christian Ethics." *Journal of Religion* 55, no. 4 (October): 470-76.

Childress, James F. 1982. *Who Should Decide?* New York: Oxford University Press.

Curran, Charles. 1973. *Politics, Medicine, and Christian Ethics.* Philadelphia: Fortress Press.

Johnson, James T., and David H. Smith, eds. 1974. *Love and Society: Essays in the Ethics of Paul Ramsey.* Missoula, Mont.: Scholars Press.

Lejeune, Jerome, with Paul Ramsey and Gerard Wright. 1984. *The Question of In Vitro Fertilization.* London: SPUC Trust.

Ramsey, Paul. 1950. *Basic Christian Ethics.* New York: Charles Scribner's Sons.

————. 1961. *War and the Christian Conscience.* Durham, N.C.: Duke University Press.

————. 1962. *Nine Modern Moralists.* Englewood Cliffs, N.J.: Prentice-Hall.

————. 1967. *Deeds and Rules in Christian Ethics.* New York: Charles Scribner's Sons.

————. 1968a. "The Case of the Curious Exception." In Ramsey and Outka 1968: 67-135.

————. 1968b. "The Morality of Abortion." In *Life or Death: Ethics and Options,* ed. Daniel H. Labby, 60-72. Seattle: University of Washington Press.

————. 1970a. *The Patient as Person.* New Haven: Yale University Press.

————. 1970b. *Fabricated Man.* New Haven: Yale University Press.

————. 1971. "The Morality of Abortion." In *Moral Problems,* ed. James Rachels. New York: Harper and Row. (A revision of Ramsey 1968b.)

————. 1973. "Abortion: A Review Article." *The Thomist* 37, no. 1 (January): 174-226.

————. 1976. "Some Rejoinders." *Journal of Religious Ethics* 4, no. 2 (Fall): 185-237.

————. 1978. *Ethics at the Edges of Life.* New Haven: Yale University Press.

Ramsey, Paul, and Gene Outka, eds. 1968. *Norm and Context in Christian Ethics.* New York: Charles Scribner's Sons.

ON JAMES M. GUSTAFSON

Can Medical Ethics Be Christian?

ALLEN VERHEY

JAMES M. Gustafson was one of the first theologians to turn attention to medical ethics in the sixties. He was involved in discussions about medical ethics from the very beginning of that decade at Yale. And in the seventies he was also one of the first theologians publicly to lament the fact that although persons trained in theology had begun to comment frequently on issues in medical ethics, they seldom made explicit reference to theological traditions or to religious convictions (1978). He acknowledged that there were sometimes good reasons for silence about theological convictions in such commentary, but he more vigorously pointed out good reasons to lament this silence. Chief among these was the simple truth that faithful members of religious communities want to live and die and work and care with faithful integrity, not just with impartial rationality.

Gustafson's lament was echoed by many and signaled renewed attention to the relevance of theological traditions and religious convictions to medical ethics. But if one agrees that theological affirmations are relevant to issues in medical ethics, then it becomes important to think carefully about *how* theological affirmations should be brought to bear upon the powers and problems of medicine. This essay attends to that question by examining the work of James M. Gustafson as a possible model for theological reflection about medical ethics. It first analyzes his proposal of a method for relating theology to medical ethics; it then looks at some of his specific theological affirmations and their consequences in medical morality; and finally it examines some ways his method and convictions restrain and sustain his casuistry, his reflection on concrete cases and issues.

My admiration for Gustafson's moral, theological, and pastoral sensitivities I acknowledge at the outset, if only in recognition of a point Gustafson often makes, that affections inform and qualify analysis. Even so, for those who take seriously the issues of Gustafson's work, some critical response is requisite.

Gustafson's Proposal

Can medical ethics be Christian? The question is borrowed from Gustafson's *Can Ethics Be Christian?* (1975b). He answers there that ethics, including medical ethics, can be Christian because "religion *qualifies* morality" (1975b: 173).

To understand this claim, it may be helpful to define some terms (see Gustafson 1975a: 3-15). *Theology* is an intellectual discipline that reflects upon the dimension of human experience denoted "religious," that is, upon the sense of an ultimate power (or powers) that sustains and bears down upon human persons and the world. It attempts to determine "what qualities and characteristics can be appropriately attributed to the ultimate power, what purposes and intentions can be plausibly claimed for it, and what its relations are to the world" (1975a: 7). *Christian theology*, then, is simply such an intellectual discipline undertaken within the context of the faith and tradition of the Christian community, where the experience of an ultimate power is nurtured and informed by the memory of certain religiously significant events, concepts, and symbols.

Ethics, too, is an intellectual discipline that reflects upon a dimension of human experience, the dimension of human experience denoted "moral." It attempts "to analyze the necessary conditions for moral activity" and "to indicate normatively what moral principles and values ought to govern human action" (1975a: 13). *Medical ethics* is simply the ethics that restricts its interest to the moral dimensions of human action in the arena of medicine.

The "*religious* qualification of moral experience" (1975a: 13) occurs when there is an awareness that one acts not only in response to other persons and other actions but also in response to the ultimate power that sustains and bears down upon human persons and the world.

And the *"theological* qualification of *ethics"* (1975a: 13) occurs when account is taken of the ultimate power's character, purposes, and relations to the world and of their significance for analyzing the necessary conditions for moral action or for indicating the principles and values that ought to govern it.

"Religion *qualifies* morality." This claim distinguishes Gustafson not only from those who claim that ethics cannot be (and should not be) Christian (on the basis, for example, of an identification of "the moral point of view" with an impartial and purely rational perspective), but also from those who claim that ethics can be (and should be) Christian either because Christian ethics is simply identical with universal and rational principles of morality or because Christian ethics is absolutely contrasted with disciplined reflection on *human* experience by being knowledge given exclusively by revelation. (See 1975b: 170-72.)

Because religion *qualifies* morality, a Christian ethic, including a Christian medical ethic, must undertake two tasks: it must come to terms with and relate itself to the dimension of *human* experience denoted "moral," and it must "qualify" that experience in the light of religious experience of the character and purposes of God. Gustafson consistently rebukes the failure to undertake either of these two tasks. He criticizes the natural law tradition of much Roman Catholic commentary on medical ethics for its assumption that there is an autonomous and natural moral order that can be known and applied on the basis of reason alone and to which an explicitly Christian word may be added as ultimate authorization or extra obligation (1978: 387). He is prepared to honor that tradition for the attention it gives to "natural" morality, but he rebukes it for neglecting the necessary and radical reorientation of morality in the light of religious experience and Christian convictions. He also criticizes the position of those confessional Protestants who interpret technology, the cultural ethos, and contemporary institutions as demonic powers against which the Christian must announce the good news and the claims of the gospel (1978: 389-90). He is prepared to honor their "radically prophetic stance" (1978: 389), but he rebukes them for their inattention to the real situation of human choice with its limitations and ambiguities, for their failure to own responsibility in a world rightly and easily under prophetic censure.[1]

---

1. The question of the relation of theology and ethics is analogous to the question of the relation of Christ and culture examined by Gustafson's teacher, H. Richard

The proposal that religion qualifies morality can be defended, of course, not only by appeals to the human experiences denoted "moral" and "religious" but also by appeals to certain theological convictions. "Drawing deeply on the Reformed tradition," Gustafson affirms that God is related to the world as Creator, Sustainer, Judge, and Redeemer (1981: 193, 235-51).[2] Because God is related to the world as Creator and Sustainer — and not just in some distant and forsaken past — nature and the "natural" human experience of morality may not be ignored or forsaken. Because God is related to the world as Judge, the "fault" that runs through human loyalties, valuations, perceptions, and actions (1981: 294) may not be forgotten; a Christian ethic may not simply be identified with the "natural" experience of morality or simply added to it. Because God is related to the world as Redeemer, a radical reorientation of human moral experience is called for: a radical reorientation *of natural morality* because the relation of God as Creator may not be ignored nor the human experience of God's creative and sustaining power dismissed, and a *radical reorientation* of natural morality because of the capacity (and tendency) of human beings to "turn inward" (1981: 306), to be motivated by self-interest alone.

Since religion qualifies *morality,* it is obviously important to identify the morality to be qualified. If, for example, moral experience were simply an experience of being obliged to obey certain laws or to seek certain ends, then a Christian ethic would have to come to terms with and somehow qualify them. Or if moral experience were simply an

---

Niebuhr (1951). Gustafson himself acknowledged the connection between his proposal that "religion *qualifies* morality" and Niebuhr's ideal type, "Christ the Transformer of Culture" (see Gustafson 1981: 192-93). Gustafson also critiques the alternative models in Niebuhr's typology as methods for Christian reflection concerning medical ethics. Niebuhr's criticism of the "Christ above Culture" model is paralleled by Gustafson's rejection of the natural law approach of some Roman Catholic commentary on medical ethics. And Niebuhr's criticism of the "Christ against Culture" model is followed by Gustafson's rejection of the prophetic rhetoric of some confessional Protestants.

If Gustafson's criticisms of other methods are revealing, so are others' criticisms of Gustafson. Both Richard McCormick (1981: 310-11) and Stanley Hauerwas (1978) echoed Gustafson's lament that theological affirmations seldom informed medical ethics, but McCormick urged Gustafson in the direction of recognizing the integrity of "natural" moral reasoning, and Hauerwas urged him in the direction of emphasizing the particularity of Christian convictions and ethics over against culture.

2. On Gustafson's "preference for the Reformed tradition" as well as his problems with certain aspects of it, see 1981: 157-93.

experience of radical freedom, as put forth by existentialists, then a Christian ethic would have to come to terms with such autonomy and somehow qualify the subjective authenticity that makes a decision valid. Gustafson's account of morality, however — both of the conditions necessary for moral experience and of the reflection required in deciding what to do — is considerably more complex than those.

The moral experience to be qualified by religion is always the experience of particular persons in specific circumstances and related to other persons, institutions, laws, or events in mutual dependence. It is in the context of this interdependence that one experiences moral obligation. The relationships are not static: there are possibilities for responding to actions upon one and for initiating actions toward another, for altering the relationship, for reforming oneself, for influencing the other, but the possibilities, too, are limited. They are limited by the determinate features of the agent, of the circumstances, and of "the other." These real but limited possibilities provide the occasion for an agent both to act and to reflect concerning such action (1975b: 2-14).

This account of morality requires Gustafson to focus on the agents when he looks at specific cases and to insist that these agents be understood both in terms of the ways they express personal histories accumulated through nature, time, and communities and in terms of the freedom they have to determine a future without being wholly determined by nature or history (1981: 288; 1968b: 93; see also 1975b: 25-47; 1981: 281-93). On Gustafson's model of agency, various dependencies and interdependencies limit and provide the genuine options people have to affect courses of events in accordance with ideals and intentions. Human rationality and freedom are not denied, but neither are they simply contrasted to needs, desires, "natural" affections, and determinate features of our biology, of our social and cultural conditioning, or of our history and communities. To be sure, human valuing requires critical reflection about conflicting values and alternative objects of desire, but rationality exists and is exercised in intimate relation to affectivity. And freedom, on this account, is much more limited than often claimed, limited "to marshall and direct realities which exist prior to our choices and actions" (1981: 290).

Gustafson's distance from moral theories which single-mindedly emphasize autonomy should be plain. "Certainly it is correct to respect [persons'] capacity for agency," Gustafson says, "but persons are more than their capacity for agency. We must also respect their bodily natures, and we have responsibilities to see that they are not deprived of necessities. We are to respect persons not merely as individuals but as 'members one of another' in their communities" (1981: 291).

To focus on the agent, then, is not to limit one's vision to the moral fiction of an autonomous individual (or noumenal self) but to attend to the various dependencies and interdependencies that provide and limit choices; it is to focus on the person in time and in community. Correlatively, Gustafson proposes an "interactional model of society" (1981: 293) that recognizes both the formation of the self and its choices by society and the alteration of social orders and relations and courses of events by human agency. He admits that there is in the interactional model no simple way to determine whether in particular cases "the common good" should take precedence (as in organic theories of society) or "individual rights" (as in contractual theories).

This account of agency appeals to moral experience, but it is also backed by theological affirmations, specifically by the Reformed tradition's appreciation for "the limitations upon human capacities to determine human destiny, and the destiny of the world" (1981: 186). And it is in terms of this model of agency that religious convictions can qualify agents' understanding of themselves, of their circumstances, and of their possible actions.

The morality to be "qualified" may be described not only in terms of moral agency but also in terms of reflection concerning what ought to be done and why. In Gustafson's account moral reflection is not simply an application of rules or principles, nor simply a calculation of consequences, nor simply an exercise of a moral "sense." Moral reflection is a complex human enterprise of *discernment.* The "common elements in all moral discernment" (1968a: 23) include the perspective from which one interprets the meaning of human experience, the characteristics of the person discerning (including the dispositions, attitudes, and affections of the person), and the fundamental principles and values that are held to govern conduct. Discernment — and each of its elements — should be qualified by the experience of the presence and power of God and by reflection concerning God's character, purposes, and relations with the world.

One implication of this account of discernment is that neither an ethic of virtue nor an ethic of obligation is alone adequate to the human experience of making moral decisions. Both the formation of worthy character and the identification of certain normative principles are features of morality and of morality as qualified by Christianity. A second implication is that both radical relativism and absolute certainty fail to "fit" the human experience of discernment. Principles and values are knowable and applicable, and some things "are always wrong" (1981: 340), but in the concrete limitations of choice in complex circumstances there is often no absolute moral certainty. Values and principles do not fall into neat hierarchies; genuine values and principles can genuinely conflict. The final discernment is not a strict deduction from a single principle but something more like a "moment of perception that sees the parts in relation to a whole, expresses sensibilities as well as reasoning, and is made in the conditions of human finitude" (1981: 338). Both an appreciation for principles and an acknowledgment of complexity and ambiguity are fitting to the human experience of discernment. A Christian ethic does not rescue us from ambiguity, but it should qualify our experience of ambiguity along with our perspective on "the whole" to which we are related, our sensibilities along with our principles.

Religion qualifies morality. This statement forces attention not only to the morality to be qualified but to religious experience and to theological reflection concerning religious experience as well. Before we consider the particular theological affirmations Gustafson would bring to bear on medical ethics, we need to consider the licenses he would grant and the limits he would impose for making them.

The place to begin is again with experience, for human experience is prior to reflection upon it (1981: 115-29). Religious experience is "not unnatural" (1981: 134). The power and presence of God can evoke certain "senses" even in those who do not name God "I am" and, for that matter, even in those who deny that God is. Gustafson calls these senses a "natural piety" (1980: 758; see also 1981: 129-36) and describes them as senses of dependence upon and gratitude for those on whom we rely, senses of obligation and remorse in response to the orderings of life and our failure to conform to them, senses of the possibilities and direction for human action. These senses are evoked in human experience of "others" but seem also to invoke the "muted honoring of Another about which not much is said" (1980a: 750). The "step" of Christianity is to experience and acknowledge the power and presence of the God whom Jesus called Father, to experience and acknowledge this God as the one who — through diverse experiences and diverse others — evokes the senses of dependence and gratitude, obligation and remorse, possibility and direction, and as the one to whom reverence and respect are finally due. Such piety with its "religious affections" qualifies morality; it requires that life "be conformed to that ordering activity of God which we cannot fully know" (1980a: 759).

Theological affirmations, of course, attempt to say what we *can* know about God. Although what we can know about God should be brought to bear on how we think about morality, including medical morality, Gustafson is wary of the "excessive certainty" (1984: 7; see also 1991: 89) with which some theologians talk of God and of God's intentions. He points out that any particular theology is a "selective retrieval" of elements in the "great variety" of biblical and traditional claims (1981: 141). His modesty about knowledge of God shows up as well in his openness to testing theological affirmations not only by their coherence with the tradition but also, and fundamentally, by their coherence with human experience and in the light of other areas of knowledge. What is said theologically may not be dishonest to one's own experience (1980a: 759) or "incongruous" with the best knowledge of the world we have from other sources of knowledge, including the human sciences (1981: 136-50, 257). And his caution concerning how thoroughly we can know God shows up, finally, in the priority he gives (in both the method and the substance of his argument) to the affirmation of God's transcendence.

The first and fundamental theological affirmation is the transcendence of God: it is God who is God, and not we ourselves. There are a number of important implications of making God's transcendence central. First, because he affirms God's transcendence, Gustafson refuses to render religion instrumental to human moral (or prudential) ends. It is not that he denies the "utility" of religion, but he insists that persons are to serve God's purposes and not God our purposes. "In Christian experience . . . the religious dimensions have priority over the moral. The existence of God is not posited to have an ultimate ground for morality; rather the reality of God is experienced, and this experience requires morality . . ." (1975b: 173; see also 1980a: 755-56; 1981: 16-25).

Second, his affirmation of God's transcendence leads Gustafson to reject the anthropocentrism of much of Western philosophical and theological morality. While it is human persons who measure morally, it is God who is the measure of things morally (1980a: 755; 1981: 81-82). The whole creation and the other creatures in it must be seen in terms of their relation to God rather than simply in terms of their instrumental value for human persons. Accordingly, Gustafson consistently directs moral attention to the larger whole of which humanity is a part and to the larger purpose of God within which our finite purposes and measuring must be assessed.

Third, Gustafson calls for piety to form the intention to relate to all things in ways appropriate to their relation to God (1975b: 66, 75, 76; 1981: 158, 227; 1984: 146, 275). Of course, if that call is to be meaningful, if the intention is to be carried out, then the transcendent God cannot be altogether unknowable, an empty cipher behind or beyond all human attempts to describe God.

According to Gustafson the character and purposes of the transcendent God are not unknowable, even if they are not fully and exhaustively knowable. The transcendent God is not a totally unknown God, even if God can be known only by analogy.[3] There is, however, no simple understanding of God or of God's purpose without the risk of absolutizing a particular understanding rather than God. There are "no divinely initiated or infallibly revealed prescriptions of proper actions" (1984: 275), "no precise moral blueprint in nature" (1984: 275), not even in the patterns of the interdependencies of life. But experience of the power of God and reflection about God and God's purposes on the basis of scripture, tradition, nature, and the interdependencies of life can provide "indications of points to be taken into account in making personal and social choices" and set such choices within a "larger context" (1984: 275). The purposes of God that we do know, however, are multiple, not single. To be sure, the purposes of God can be summarized in a generalized conception like "God intends the well-being of the creation" (1975a: 18), but such summaries will involve unavoidably complex and not simple notions. A plurality of values can be justified by what we can know of God, and these cannot be forced into a neat

---

3. Gordon Kaufmann distinguished a "teleological" model of God's transcendence, leading to analogies of being, and a "personalistic" model of God's transcendence, leading to analogies of agency (*God the Problem*, cited in Gustafson 1981: 264). Gustafson rejected not just Kaufmann's choice of the personalistic model (as Kant's "noumenal self" writ large) but the bifurcation itself. It is worth remembering that Gustafson's account of agency refused to make the split between "noumenal self" and "phenomenal self." It is not so much that Gustafson rejects the analogy of agency as that he would develop it more circumspectly (1981: 270), in ways more attentive to and appreciative of what might be called God's "phenomenal self," the presence of his power in nature, in history, in communities, in those determinate features of our existence which make agency possible as well as limit it.

set of priorities that will eliminate genuine dilemmas or the tragedy of choosing between evils or incompatible goods (1969: 101-4).

Can medical ethics be Christian? Yes, but it is evidently a methodologically complex matter. Gustafson relates the anecdote that, when he once described his work to a moral philosopher, the philosopher was prompted to say, "It may be easier to find out what's right than to find out how Christians should go about deciding what's right" (1975b: 143). The remark is a cogent one. Gustafson's response is that the observation vitiates the undertaking of a Christian ethic only if the religious dimensions of experience are not to be taken seriously. If they are to be taken seriously, then the relations of persons and communities to the power that sustains them and stands over against them provide a context for their relating to all else, including medical morality.

Gustafson's Theological Claims and Medical Ethics

In this section I undertake to identify at least some of the theological affirmations Gustafson makes and the ways they "qualify" perspective, dispositions, intentions, and judgments in medical ethics. Gustafson's 1975 Pere Marquette Theology Lecture, *The Contributions of Theology to Medical Ethics*, provides a starting place.

There Gustafson makes three theological affirmations: "God intends the well-being of the creation" (1975a: 18). "God is both the ordering power that preserves and sustains the well-being of the creation and the power that creates new possibilities for well-being in events of nature and history" (1975a: 19). "Humans are finite and 'sinful' agents whose actions have a large measure of power to determine whether the well-being of the creation is sustained or fulfilled" (1975a: 22). These affirmations represent a selective retrieval of dimensions of experience as reflected upon in the Jewish and Christian communities. Gustafson does not defend the selection of these affirmations in the lecture; rather, they are simply brought to bear upon medical ethics in ways that cohere with his method. Inferences are drawn that "qualify" morality, including perspective, dispositions, and intentions.

"God intends the well-being of the creation." That affirmation qualifies one's moral perspective, in the first place, by providing a reason for being moral (1975a: 25). The point is not that without this affirmation, without "God," there is no reason for being moral, only that this affirmation does provide a reason for being moral and, for those who share such an affirmation, a reason of the utmost seriousness and stringency. It is *God* who intends the well-being of the creation, God who sustains it and creates new possibilities for it, and we are responsible finally to God, also morally. Morality is authorized not merely on the basis of human self-fulfillment and not merely on the basis of rationality; it is authorized by the affective and rational affirmation that God intends the well-being of the creation.

The theological qualification of medical morality occurs, moreover, not just at the level of response to the question "Why be moral?" Precisely because theology qualifies morality at that level, it qualifies it everywhere. The moral point of view is neither justified nor constituted solely by pure rationality. Because it can be justified by theological affirmations, it should be qualified by theological affirmations. If the power that bears down on us and sustains us were indifferent to values, then theological affirmations could not supply a reason for being moral; but because that power is not indifferent, because God intends *well-being,* theological affirmations bear on morality itself (1975a: 26, 30). "Theology does not only provide 'ultimate grounds' for morality; the morality that it grounds is qualified by the theological beliefs" (1975b: 174).

The affirmation that God intends the well-being of *the whole creation* restrains and chastens the anthropocentric perspective that has shaped the vision of most Western philosophical (and religious) thought. The moral perspective, including the moral perspective in the arena of medicine, is qualified by that affirmation; the "qualified" moral perspective includes the whole creation and its flourishing as its horizon. Humanity and its flourishing are a part of that, to be sure, and there is a "qualitative distinction" (1975a: 65) between the way human beings and other species are related to God, but human well-being is not the only thing that captures our attention when we look at things from this perspective. The "common good" is enlarged to include more than our immediate and human neighbors, and the "totality" to be kept in view is not only the individual's embodied self or some human community but the total creation. From such a perspective one could see the moral possibility of sometimes overriding (but never sweepingly disregarding) individual rights and claims to well-being for the sake of a more inclusive well-being (1975a: 33-35).

The moral perspective is qualified as well by inferences from the affirmation that God is the power that both sustains well-being and creates new possibilities for well-being. Because God is the power that *sustains* well-being, the point of view is conservative. Those principles, values, institutions, sanctions, and other features of our relations and circumstances that work to preserve and conserve life and well-being are to be respected and themselves preserved (1975a: 36-37). But because God is the power that *creates new possibilities* of well-being, the point of view is open to the alteration of values. This theological affirmation qualifies the perspective so that we are able to see that some changes in principles, values, rules, and practices may be changes for the better (1975a: 37-54).

These theological affirmations qualify not only moral perspective but also the moral attitudes, the dispositions, the readiness to act and react in certain ways, in short, the character, of the moral agent. Gustafson elucidates as examples three attitudes: respect for life, openness to new possibilities, and self-criticism.

The attitude of respect for life, the readiness to protect, sustain, and nurture it, is inferred from the intention of God for well-being because life is a necessary condition for well-being. God's creative and sustaining powers are similarly warrants for the readiness to receive and respect life as a gift and as a good.

Because God intends the well-being of the whole creation, of course, this "respect for life is to be directed toward all living things" (1975a: 78). There can be no readiness to exploit and destroy animals or plants for the satisfaction of immediate human interests. This attitude tempers destructive intrusions into nature; it is ready to demand "that good reasons must be given to intervene in the processes of biological life" (1975a: 59); and it will feel anguish at the costs borne by the rest of the creation for the sake of human comfort and well-being. The attitude does not resolve such conflicts of value, however, or deny that intervention into biological processes for the sake of human well-being is ever justified. Theological affirmations warrant an attitude of respect for life, but they also prevent the absolutizing of this attitude (or value) (1975a: 60-63; 1969). There are occasions in which physical life may be (mournfully) sacrificed for other values.

An attitude of "openness" is warranted by the theological affirmation that God is a creative power establishing new possibilities of well-being. This attitude includes the courage to take risks in order to realize emerging possibilities for well-being in developments in nature and in history. This openness coexists in some tension with other attitudes, which are also theologically warranted: the disposition to conserve present well-being, for example, and the attitude of respect, the "primitive feeling of co-humanity that resists turning persons into means rather than ends" (1975a: 65). The attitude of openness stands at risk of licensing care-less human interventions and exploration unless checked by these other attitudes and by principles like "informed consent" (1975a: 63, 66), but without openness and courage, dispositions to conserve present values and to respect persons can become "dogmatic and idolatrous" (1975a: 63). Without openness we will miss new opportunities God provides.

The third attitude is "self-criticism." It is warranted by the third affirmation, that human persons are finite and sinful agents with powers to determine whether the well-being of creation is sustained and fulfilled. The recognition of finiteness and sinfulness follows reflection upon the religious senses of dependence and repentance, evoked by the transcendent God who is Creator and Judge (1975a: 67-74; also 1977). Recognition of our finiteness readies us to be cautious about medical interventions, for example, about genetic engineering or psychosurgery. We cannot foresee all the consequences of our action, and we are dependent upon determinate and limited resources. Recognition of our sinfulness readies us to be careful about our tendency to secure our own interests or the interests of our group or species at the cost of the well-being of others, for example, in research.

These attitudes establish dispositions to act and react in certain ways, but they do not tell us what precisely to do in particular contexts. They form and inform discernment, but they do not render decision unnecessary. When specific questions of conduct arise, so do judgments and justifications. That brings us to the theological qualification of direction or intention.

The theological affirmations and the moral point of view coherent with them should also form and inform certain intentions in one's life and conduct concerning medicine. The first theological affirmation, of course, articulates a certain *telos,* or end, that ought to govern our conduct: the well-being of creation. It is, however, a very general intention, requiring specification.

The specification of this *telos,* however, is a complex matter. Many "goods" are involved in the well-being of the creation, and they do not fall into simple hierarchies or pleasant harmonies. Theological affirmations do not provide a complete specification of "the well-being of the whole creation." The third affirmation, however, points us to how and why it should be attempted. The finiteness and sinfulness of human agents make absolute moral certitude in complex circumstances impossible, but they also render the objectivity and rational criticism enabled by principles and rules important (1968b: 257-58). We cannot presume to know or reproduce the precise shape of divine governance, but we can pay precise and thorough attention to the patterns and processes of interdependence of life in the world and to the possibilities for well-being they provide and limit, also in medical care and research.

Physical life, for example, is an important, indeed indispensable, element of well-being; but it may not be considered an absolute value, as though a neat hierarchy were within our intellectual grasp. Other values (relief from avoidable suffering, for example) must also be considered and may sometimes take moral precedence (1975a: 85-86). In such cases of tragic conflict of values physicians and patients can rely on the principles that have sustained and nurtured well-being in the past. The disposition to conserve present well-being will urge that rules and policies formulated out of past experience and reflection ought to be obeyed. But the disposition of openness requires us to listen to good reasons that the case is an exception or that the rules should be changed (1975a: 87-90).

Theological affirmations do not provide a complete specification of the well-being of the whole creation. Since God is a power creating new possibilities of well-being, moreover, the specification of well-being will always be in a process of discovery. "Well-being" itself is related to many natural and cultural factors, and it must be specified in relation to those factors, not once and for all (1975a: 90-92).[4]

---

4. Again Gustafson's criticisms of others are quite revealing. During the course of the Pere Marquette lecture Gustafson responds to the work of a number of Christian moral theologians. He criticizes the tradition of Roman Catholic casuistry both for its moral certitude about a harmony of ends neatly packaged in a hierarchy and for its conservative attitude to changes in values or technology. He criticizes Paul Ramsey for his conservative posture, for his lack of openness to new possibilities of well-being. He criticizes Joseph Fletcher for his utilitarianism, for his reduction of the goods to be sought to happiness, and for his confidence that tragic choices can be avoided. He criticizes Paul Lehmann for relying on sympathetic imagination rather than struggling to articulate the goods involved in well-being and their relations. He is sympathetic with Karl Rahner's position but criticizes him, along with most theological and philosophical

Theology qualifies the fundamental orientation of a person's life, therefore, but it can qualify judgments about conduct only indirectly, only through the process of discernment used to reach them. "From the standpoint of immediate practicality, the contribution of theology is not great" (1975a: 94). In spite of that modest conclusion, however, the three theological affirmations have qualified perspective, dispositions, and intentions in ways that may not logically entail any particular action but which nevertheless situate that action and reflection about it in the broader context of our response to the transcendent power. The "immediate practicality" of Gustafson's method and theology will, moreover, be the focus of the next section as we turn attention to Gustafson's casuistry, his use of theological affirmations in analyzing specific ethical cases.

Three observations must yet be made. First, Gustafson assumes and calls for communities of moral discourse and discernment. Such communities are necessary as a corrective for our finiteness and sinfulness and as an exemplification of the interdependence that is part of our dependence upon God. Our point of view, attitudes, and understanding of well-being can be less partial within the correction of moral discourse (1975a: 74-75, 92) and can be qualified by the Christian tradition and the religious experience of others within the church as a community of moral discourse and discernment (see 1970b: 83-96; 1984: 316-19).

Second, Gustafson identifies a variety of forms of moral discourse: prophetic, narrative, ethics, and public policy discourse (1988, 1990). Each is legitimate and important, but none is sufficient. Prophetic discourse uses the language of indictment and the allure of a utopian vision to identify root problems and to evoke a deep moral response. Narrative discourse uses the language of story to sustain the moral identity of a community and its members, to shape character into something coherent with the story, and to affect the way agents see and interpret the

---

moralists, for his anthropocentrism, for his inattention to the well-being of the whole creation. In each case the criticism is not only moral but theological. Rahner (and most of the tradition) has limited the well-being intended by God to human well-being, failing to attend (both affectively and intellectually) to the well-being of the whole creation. Ramsey and the natural law tradition have failed to attend to God as the power creating new possibilities for well-being. Fletcher and others have failed to acknowledge the finitude and sinfulness of human agents and the plurality of goods involved in the *telos* of well-being.

world and the possibilities for action within it. Ethical discourse refers to philosophical modes of argument and analysis, and it typically attempts to justify decisions on the basis of universal (or at least widely shared) principles and values. Policy discourse, finally, is the discourse not of external observers but of persons with responsibility and power who must attend to very particular circumstances that both enable and limit the possibilities of action. Different vocations in any community of moral discourse, including the church, will lead to different people utilizing one or another of these four forms primarily. Prophetic discourse and narrative discourse may be closer to the language of scripture and may seem to a Christian community more "natural," but churches — and public discourse, too — "need greater communication between persons who use primarily each of these forms" (1988: 53).

Third, Gustafson appreciates and qualifies the moral significance of the "professions," including the medical profession. The medical professional possesses not only technical knowledge but also certain competence in "practical reason," in making judgments about specific courses of action; the medical professional has a particular identity and is under certain social controls that are partly limiting and that sustain legitimate expectations; and the medical professional is "service oriented" (1982: 506-8). To construe the profession in the light of religious experience as a "calling" *qualifies* it, most notably by confirming and sustaining the deeply moral motives of service that frequently lead people into the profession and by enlarging the profession's vision of the ends to be served (1982: 509-12). So a physician, although "primarily concerned with the immediate needs of the patient," should also see the particular interaction with the patient as part of "a larger whole" (1984: 282). This means paying attention to others affected by care of the patient, to long-range consequences as well as immediate effects (1984: 282), and to needs of the patient that have no "technical" solution (like the need to assess the possibilities and limitations of their circumstances and the need of the lonely or despairing or dying for "company" [1984: 208]).

Gustafson's Casuistry

Whenever Gustafson has turned his attention to concrete issues and cases in medical ethics, the results have been worthy of both his pastoral and his scholarly sensitivities. His article on abortion (1970a), for example, demonstrates both methodological consistency and a pastoral identity. In it Gustafson discusses a case of pregnancy due to rape.

He begins with a consideration of the agent and her circumstances, the determinate conditions that limit and provide the opportunities for reflection and judgment, not with rules to be applied deductively to conduct. His account of the case is not that of an external judge; it is rather that of a counselor attempting to understand the position of the person who has to assume responsibility for action. He rejects the legal model of applying laws to cases and instead exercises discernment, interpreting both the situation and the rules in their larger context. He refuses to reduce the relevant data either to the fact that there are no physiological difficulties or to the fact that the pregnancy has its origin in sexual violence, and he refuses to reduce the relevant values to the single principle of respect for life. Other data are relevant, as are broader concerns of well-being. He insists that "the case" not be limited to the relations of doctor and woman and fetus at the time of pregnancy but include a broader range of relationships and interdependencies over a longer period of time. He rejects the rationalistic morality that "reduces individuals" to "abstract cases" (1970a: 105) and that dismisses the historical formation of character and choices; instead, he insists on attention to and appreciation for the determinate features of this woman's life. Finally, he insists that moral advice neither simply apply a "natural law" (which might be ultimately grounded in Christian convictions) nor merely express one's intuition; the advice should nurture and sustain the agent's capacity to exercise a discernment qualified by Christian affirmations.[5]

All of this is consistent, of course, with what we have seen of Gustafson's method, his concern for the agent's perspective, his emphasis on the phenomenal self, historically and socially formed, his appreciation of a variety of goods not easily harmonized or brought into

---

5. Gustafson also distinguishes his method from the typical Protestant reliance upon a renewed sensitivity and upon renewed human capacities to see "what God is doing" (as seen, for example, in the work of Paul Lehmann). This approach, too, presupposes a kind of moral certitude unavailable to finite and sinful agents. The possibilities of absolute moral certitude removed, the same finitude and sinfulness render traditional Roman Catholic casuistry presumptuous and typical Protestant approaches slothful. Finitude and sinfulness make rational deliberation both limited and morally necessary.

hierarchical relationship, his concern for character as well as obligation, his emphasis on broadening perspective, his "transformationist" position on bringing theology to bear on the morality of individual moral agents and on the elements of discernment.

Gustafson's own discernment in this case is self-consciously qualified by Christian affirmations. One theological affirmation here is that "God wills the creation, preservation, reconciliation, and redemption of human life" (1970a: 113). This affirmation qualifies one's perspective: life — with all its dependencies and interdependencies — is seen as a gift. It qualifies dispositions: the affirmation forms a readiness to respect and cherish human life. And it qualifies intentions: human life is to be protected and nurtured, and the conditions for its flourishing are to be sought. But, once again, this is a complex directive. The goods of human life are many and not always in harmony. They do not neatly fall into a hierarchy of values. The acknowledgment that human persons are finite and sinful agents implies the impossibility of moral certitude, the necessity of a perspective that is both conservative and open to the possibilities of well-being for the woman, and the appropriateness of attitudes of both openness and self-criticism.

Gustafson's discerning judgment follows a careful analysis of the social and historical context of the case. It is reached on the basis of principles that provide some specificity to the fundamental intention: Life is ordinarily to be preserved. The lives of the powerless are especially to be protected. There are exceptions when other goods conflict. Examples of exceptions are "medical indications," "social indications," and pregnancies that occur as a result of sexual crime.

Obviously, Gustafson cannot treat these as rules to be juridically applied. He cannot assume, for example, that abortion is morally legitimate in every case of rape or that it is morally impermissible in every case not treated by these exceptions. One is led to suppose, for example, that Gustafson would counsel against abortion if this victim of rape had the resources of a community that could be relied upon to sustain and support her. The principles and their exceptions, however, do provide a basis for rational deliberation, and on this basis Gustafson affirms the moral propriety of abortion in this instance.

He insists, however, that such a "judgment" not conclude the relation to the woman. She deserves more than a "legal" justification. As a person — if she agrees with the judgment — she needs and deserves to understand why her case is an exception. Moreover, she needs access to other resources — medical resources, financial resources, social and moral resources — and it is the moralist's obligation to attend to these as well. The concern is not simply the discrete moment and the particular relations of woman, doctor, and fetus; the concern is rather the woman's well-being over a longer period of time and in a broader network of relations, and the moralist's responsibilities must be consonant with these extended concerns.

Another example of Gustafson's casuistry is his response (1973) to the famous Johns Hopkins case. An infant with Down's syndrome and duodenal atresia (closure of the duodenum) was allowed to die because the parents refused consent for a procedure to correct the atresia. Gustafson carefully analyzes the family setting, the legal setting, and the hospital setting. He is concerned that the moralist not simply render a judicial decision on the basis of rules and principles rationally known and deductively applied to a narrowly circumscribed case. Instead, he focuses on the agents, and he attempts to understand their perspectives and the circumstances that limit and present the real possibilities of action. He works his way finally to "qualify" the agents' understanding of themselves, of their circumstances, and of the possible and appropriate action. In this essay, however, he does not first rehearse any theological affirmations and move from them to inferences about perspectives, attitudes, and intentions. He offers his conclusion that the surgery ought to have been done and the grounds for the conclusion. The grounds are the assignment of different weight to two things: the desires of the parents are given less weight, and the claims of the infant to life are given more. He defends this assignment of the values of parental desires and infant claims by appealing to what we have called "natural piety," explicitly by appealing to the senses of obligation and dependence and their relationship in our experience in families (1984: 164-76). Parents experience and sense obligation — and obligation not simply contingent upon desires — in the very dependency of their children upon them (1973: 550). The family is a "school for piety and morality" (1984: 173), for the senses of dependence, gratitude, obligation, remorse, possibility, and direction that are so fundamental to Gustafson's approach. Life in families should be enough to remind us that we are not as radically autonomous as some moral theories claim and that happiness is not what the moral life is all about. In the relationship of dependence, the dependents make a claim on those on whom they depend. Parents sense that — and that the obligation is not

48

contingent upon parental desires to fulfill it. Moreover, the relationship of dependence exists in the child's relations to the physician, too, and the physicians can and should sense that they have obligations to the child and that the obligation is not contingent upon parental desires that they fulfill it.[6]

The complexity of some neonatal cases, of course, must not be overlooked. Gustafson acknowledges that neither parent nor physician would be obliged to keep a "monstrosity" alive. The value of physical life is not an absolute value, even if it is indispensable for other goods of life, and the other goods are complex, not simple. So Gustafson raises the question, "Why would I draw the line on a different side of mongolism than the physicians did?" (1973: 554), and he responds by acknowledging that, although reasons can be given, the reasons cannot be separated neatly from other elements of discernment, including perspective and attitudes.

The exceptions to the presumption of the duty to preserve life cannot be neatly spelled out. To make such exceptions simply on the basis of intelligence alone, however, is to be unheeding of the richness and variety of human life and human goods (1984: 274). And to make them merely in order to avoid suffering is also simplistic; suffering should sometimes be borne for the sake of benefits to others, especially when the suffering is "bearable." Here Gustafson does appeal explicitly to religious convictions and to the obligation to love the neighbor, to seek the well-being of the other even at the cost of inconvenience or suffering to oneself. These considerations, of course, do not tell us where the line is to be drawn precisely, but by their formation of perspective, dispositions, and intentions, they do lead Gustafson to draw the line "on a different side of mongolism." To attempt to draw a line neatly around all the cases of permissible neglect of neonates would violate the limits that Gustafson's method imposes, for an exhaustive and neat hierarchy of goods is beyond human competence, essentially reductive of the variety of human goods, and a denial of the tragic character of many moral choices.

6. Gustafson (1984: 314) adds, "The dependence of the infant on the care of others implies that *if* the intention to have it die is morally justifiable, then for the sake not of the agent, but the recipient, it would be morally permissible to intervene actively to hasten its death." He grants, however, that from his perspective it would be necessary to consider longer-range consequences for a larger community of actively hastening the death of such an infant.

Finally, after Gustafson's decision has been defended, he announces that his view is "ultimately grounded" in religious convictions (1973: 556). Gustafson's own lament could apply to this essay, but the convictions have done more than provide "an ultimate ground." They have qualified perspective, dispositions, and intentions, and so — however mediately — judgment.

The final example of Gustafson's casuistry demonstrates the importance of discernment to the formation of policy as well as to individual choices; the issue is the allocation of biomedical research funding (1984: 253-77). Gustafson does not begin with a general principle or a theory of justice and apply it deductively. Instead he begins by analyzing the patterns of interaction within which people influence allocation decisions. Theoretical attention to a moral principle without "serious consideration of the conditions of its applicability" is "at least incomplete" (1984: 258). Gustafson insists upon appreciation for the limiting features of the political, economic, cultural, and medical contexts of decisions about funding research. Moral discernment in such contexts requires attitudes of both openness and conservation, but although they are at work in Gustafson's treatment, they are not directly commented upon. Instead he focuses on the plurality of values involved in policy choices and attempts to qualify them from his theocentric perspective. As he says, there is no "preestablished harmony of all the ends, values, and principles that are worthy of support and that are applicable to a complex policy choice" (1984: 272). Along with consideration of medical, economic, and political dimensions of choices, one must consider the moral dimensions of policy choices.

Gustafson refuses to reduce the moral dimensions of policy formation to a single principle; he says quite candidly that "the ethical writings on biomedical research which focus almost exclusively on the issues of possible violations of informed consent and similar matters are ethically shortsighted" (1984: 276). Such concerns are valid, but they must be joined to other concerns with which they may sometimes be in tension. Notions of distributive justice, of legitimate means, of weighing costs and benefits, and of the common good are all relevant — and they are all "qualified" from Gustafson's theological perspective. For example, one does not simply deduce from a theory of justice how to allocate limited funds justly; instead, at various points in the interactions concerning policy it may be possible and, if so, necessary to consider whether an allocation is reasonably fair. Consideration of costs and benefits must attend not only to the short-range costs and benefits to a few but the longer-range effects upon a larger community and, indeed, the whole creation. Similarly, the good to be sought in policy concerning allocations of funds for research should not be reduced to physical life but enlarged to other goods as well. Research will not take natural processes as sacrosanct, but no reflection about research may deny our finitude, our mortality, or our dependence upon nature. Research may serve the goods of human life and health, but no reflection about research that starts with the affirmation of God's transcendence will permit such goods to become idols.

Gustafson's reasoning about the allocation of research funding does not provide a precise moral imperative applicable to concrete policy questions, but it does enable and require discernment within the particular circumstances that limit and provide possibilities. Policy decisions, too, should be accompanied by the senses of gratitude and dependence, of obligation and remorse, of possibility and direction, that are nurtured and sustained by experience of the power and presence of God.

Response

My own perspective has been shaped by the Reformed tradition which Gustafson expresses a preference for. Gustafson's claim that religion qualifies morality, the theological convictions about God's relations to the world that are used to back it, the emphasis on the transcendence of God, the importance of piety, including the "natural piety" Calvin called the *sensus divinitatis,* the recognition of the determinacies and limitations in human life and choice — all that has its roots in the Reformed tradition, and the same tradition informs my sympathy with Gustafson on these points. Other theologians may criticize Gustafson on these methodological and substantive issues, but I won't.

I do, however, want to raise some questions about Gustafson's proposal of a method and his exercise of it. The first question concerns the morality to be qualified, and it is this: Has Gustafson done justice to the categorical prohibitions based on a respect for agency? Gustafson acknowledges that some things are "always wrong," and he grounds such categorical prohibitions in "respect for persons" (see, for example, 1984: 340), but such acknowledgment is always followed and overwhelmed by Gustafson's appreciation of the conflict of values. The

Reformed tradition, for all its emphasis on the importance of perspective and the "religious affections" and for all its modesty about the capacities of human beings to understand or to will the truly good, has generally been readier to articulate certain absolutes of "the moral law," certain categorical prohibitions that are knowable apart from consideration of "the good" and that constrain even those pursuing genuine goods. Such categorical boundaries would surely be minimal, and they would not tell us what to do in complex circumstances, but they may be part of that moral experience which Christian theology must come to terms with and somehow qualify. They might help us to identify some things we ought never do, even when what we ought to do remains ambiguous. On his own presuppositions, it seems to me, Gustafson could have carried his acknowledgment of objective moral boundaries another step and identified some of them. That would have been no small service to reflection about medical morality, even if it would not have removed complexity or the tragic conflict of goods.

Concretely, Gustafson's broadening of the "totality" to be kept in view from the embodied self to the whole creation exists in some tension with the "primitive feeling of co-humanity that resists turning persons into means rather than ends" (1975a: 33, 65). This tension, of course, is coherent with Gustafson's refusal to accept either the organic model or the contractual model of social relations; on his interactional model sometimes "individual rights" and sometimes "the common good" will take moral precedence. The point, however, is that, although Gustafson plainly does not license sweeping disregard of individual rights, he does not treat any individual rights as categorical but as values to be weighed against considerations of a broader well-being. And the question is whether that is sufficient, whether it provides adequate protection for agents, however narrowly understood agency is.

The second question concerns the qualifications of the theology to be brought to bear on morality. The Reformed tradition will applaud, of course, both the emphasis on the transcendence of God and the acknowledgment that the transcendent God is known — however partially — in nature and history and experience and scripture. Gustafson's demand, then, that theological affirmations not be incongruent with our best knowledge of nature and history should not sound strange to Calvinists. But nature and history are not the primary sources; the primary source in Reformed theology is scripture and the ways scripture has illumined the church's life and shattered the church's pretensions. The *sensus divinitatis* has often been misled by the "powers" of nature and history to idolatrous trusts and loyalties. Nature and history reflect both God's power and the mysterious human powers to withstand God. To discern the governance of God in nature or in history is therefore, as Gustafson acknowledges, a complex business, but doomed to failure without "the spectacles" of scripture, to use Calvin's idiom ([1536] 1960: I.vi.1, I.xiv.1). The question is not whether Gustafson is in principle right that theological affirmations must be congruent with our best knowledge but whether the test may be as uncritically applied.

Gustafson questions, for example, Christian eschatological affirmations (those concerning the final destiny of the world) because of the best scientific knowledge about the world's future (see 1981: 268). But God transcends nature, too. Christians were — and are — reminded of their dependence upon God by their dependence upon nature, but God is dependable even when nature is not, and God is free to act independently of nature.[7]

Eschatological affirmations have fundamentally to do with the basis and object of hope. Hope that has no basis is simply wishful thinking. Hope that has no object is merely sentimental optimism. The basis of Christian hope is not scientific predictions about nature or history. The basis of Christian hope is nature's God and history's God, not nature and history, although experiential correlates must be found in nature and in history.[8] And the object of Christian hope is the cosmic reign of God, a reign within which human persons and the nature of which they are a part flourish, a reign in which the earth will rejoice and the poor will be blessed. One hopes, of course, when these things are "not yet," when there are at least some "incongruities" with the data

---

7. This is related, of course, to Gustafson's reticence to use personal analogies for speaking of the transcendent God (explicitly in 1981: 268; see note 3). To speak of the freedom of God, however, need not be an unchastened analogy to "the noumenal self"; in the Reformed tradition the freedom of God is not the arbitrary and whimsical freedom of a neutral agent but the capacity of God to covenant and so to establish an identity to which God is faithful. That covenanting may be seen in nature (for example, Genesis 8:22; 9:12-17) and in history, but the question remains where we best learn of God's established self.

8. See Gustafson's essay "The Conditions for Hope: Reflection on Human Experience" (1971: 205-16), which places more modest and more helpful constraints on eschatological affirmations.

of nature and history; but such hope nevertheless qualifies our perspective by the horizon it gives, our intentions by the direction it gives, and our dispositions by the courage it provides to stand in spite of the "incongruities" for the sake of God's cause and future. This is admittedly sketchy, but perhaps it is enough to suggest the plausibility of using Gustafson's methodological proposal with more theological confidence than Gustafson thinks fitting (or with fewer of his "skeptical hedgings," to use a phrase from Hans Jonas's commentary [1980: 216] on Gustafson's proposal).

It might be asked, moreover, whether Gustafson himself is fully consistent with his restrictive qualifications upon theological (and especially eschatological) affirmations. That God's purpose involves the well-being of the whole creation, for example, is an affirmation that may better be made with eschatological warrants than with scientific ones. The scientific predictions on which Gustafson relies to challenge anthropocentrism, after all, hold no great promise for the ecosystem of which humans are part either. Again, that God's care is particularly sensitive to the poor and powerless, the weak and oppressed (1970a: 114), an affirmation that grounds certain moral dispositions and intentions, is an affirmation that hardly seems congruent with "natural selection." To be sure, Gustafson encompasses it within the senses of dependence and interdependence, but those senses can be, sometimes are, and — in my view — should be sustained, nurtured, and enlarged by an eschatological vision of God's blessing upon the poor and helpless.

The last word concerning Gustafson's theological contribution to medical ethics must be one of deep appreciation. Medical ethics can be Christian, and it can be that less arrogantly and more discerningly because James Gustafson insists that God will not be manipulated or denied, that God will be God (1984: 319-22).

References

Calvin, John. [1559] 1960. *Institutes of the Christian Religion*, ed. John T. McNeill, trans. Ford Lewis Battles. Philadelphia: Westminster Press.
Gustafson, James M. 1968a. "Moral Discernment in the Christian Life." In *Norm and Context in Christian Ethics*, ed. Gene H. Outka and Paul Ramsey, 17-36. New York: Charles Scribner's Sons. (Reprinted in Gustafson 1974: 99-119.)

————. 1968b. *Christ and the Moral Life.* New York: Harper and Row.

————. 1969. "The Transcendence of God and the Value of Human Life." In *Proceedings* of the 23d Annual Convention of the Catholic Theological Society of America, vol. 23, 96-108. Yonkers, N.Y.: St. Joseph's Seminary. (Reprinted in Gustafson 1971: 139-49.)

————. 1970a. "A Protestant Ethical Approach." In *The Morality of Abortion,* ed. John T. Noonan, Jr., 101-22. Cambridge, Mass.: Harvard University Press.

————. 1970b. *The Church as Moral Decision-Maker.* Philadelphia: Pilgrim Press.

————. 1971. *Christian Ethics and the Community.* Philadelphia: Pilgrim Press.

————. 1973. "Mongolism, Parental Desires, and the Right to Life." *Perspectives in Biology and Medicine* 16 (Summer): 529-57.

————. 1974. *Theology and Christian Ethics.* Philadelphia: Pilgrim Press.

————. 1975a. *The Contributions of Theology to Medical Ethics.* Milwaukee: Marquette University Press.

————. 1975b. *Can Ethics Be Christian?* Chicago: University of Chicago Press.

————. 1977. "Interdependence, Finitude, and Sin: Reflections on Scarcity." *Journal of Religion* 572 (April): 156-68.

————. 1978. "Theology Confronts Technology and the Life Sciences." *Commonweal* 105 (June 16): 386-92.

————. 1980a. "A Theocentric Interpretation of Life." *Christian Century* 30 July–6 August, 754-60.

————. 1980b. "Theology and Ethics: An Interpretation of the Agenda." In *Knowing and Valuing: The Search for Common Roots,* ed. H. Tristram Engelhardt, Jr., and Daniel Callahan, 181-202. Briarcliff Manor, N.Y.: Hastings Center, Institute for Society, Ethics and the Life Sciences.

————. 1981. *Ethics from a Theocentric Perspective, Volume One: Theology and Ethics.* Chicago: University of Chicago Press.

————. 1982. "Professions as 'Callings.'" *Social Service Review* 56 (December): 501-15.

————. 1984. *Ethics from a Theocentric Perspective, Volume Two: Ethics and Theology.* Chicago: University of Chicago Press.

————. 1988. *Varieties of Moral Discourse: Prophetic, Narrative, Ethical, and Policy.* Grand Rapids: Calvin College and Seminary, The Stob Lectures Endowment.

————. 1990. "Moral Discourse about Medicine: A Variety of Forms." *Journal of Medicine and Philosophy* 15, no. 2: 125-42.

————. 1991. "All Things in Relation to God: An Interview with James M. Gustafson." *Second Opinion* 16 (March): 80-107.

Hauerwas, Stanley. 1978. "Can Ethics Be Theological?" *Hastings Center Report* 815 (October): 47-48.

Jonas, Hans. 1980. "Response to James M. Gustafson." In *Knowing and Valuing: The Search for Common Roots,* ed. H. Tristram Engelhardt, Jr., and Daniel Callahan, 203-17. Briarcliff Manor, N.Y.: Hastings Center, Institute for Society, Ethics and the Life Sciences.

McCormick, Richard A. 1981. "Bioethics and Method: Where Do We Start?" *Theological Digest* 29 (Winter): 303-18.

Niebuhr, H. Richard. 1951. *Christ and Culture.* New York: Harper and Row.

ON STANLEY HAUERWAS

Theology, Medical Ethics, and the Church

STEPHEN E. LAMMERS

IN AN article on the Methodist faith tradition, Harold Y. Vanderpool claims that the primary impetus of early Methodism lay in its determination to be a church like the early church (1986: 317). Stanley Hauerwas continues as a faithful son of that tradition, calling the church today to be more like the early Christian community. He claims that if the modern church would be more like that community, not only would it be truer to itself but it would also be of some help to the larger world. Hauerwas goes on to argue that medicine needs to be surrounded by a community like the church so that medicine can be true to its commitments.

Giving the church a central place in his theology makes Hauerwas's theological enterprise distinctively different from that of many other theologians writing today. It obligates him to a thoroughgoing rethinking of Christian ethics. He is also among the younger of the thinkers being considered in this volume, so his position is still developing, and Hauerwas himself admits to unexplained lacunae in his arguments (see 1983: "Introduction"). His recent systematic account of Christian ethics, *The Peaceable Kingdom,* forms the basis for Parts I and II of my exposition. His writings on medicine (primarily essays, many of which predate *The Peaceable Kingdom* and have been reissued in *Suffering Presence*), along with his most recent work, *Naming the Silences: God, Medicine, and the Problem of Suffering,* are the focus of Part III. In no sense do these works exhaust the Hauerwas corpus. He has written a number of essays on war, collected in *Against the Nations: War and Survival in a Liberal Society* (1985a), and on Christian ethics — *Truthfulness and Tragedy* (1977) and *A Community of Character* (1981). His first book-length publication (1975) focused on the idea of character in theological ethics. He has also shown an interest in topics as diverse as story and theology, the Christian community, and retarded children.

I. Liberalism and Contemporary Theological Ethics

Hauerwas's approach demands that he attend to the historical circumstances in which he finds himself. We are, he claims, historical beings, bounded by the time and the place in which we live. This is as true of theology as other disciplines. We begin therefore with his account of Christian theological ethics in late twentieth-century American society, so that we can see what views Hauerwas is seeking to correct.

Hauerwas maintains that many theological ethicists often disguise the fact that what they do has any relation to theology. Like his teacher James Gustafson, Hauerwas criticizes those theologians who, in an effort to make arguments and reach conclusions accessible to anyone in this society, do theological ethics as if their Christian convictions were not important (1985c: 12). Hauerwas argues that such an approach demands that religious particularities not hold the center of attention in ethical discourse (1986b: 142) and that ethicists downplay the distinctively Christian features of their convictions. The language of the larger society that theologians then have to use in making their arguments is the language of liberalism. Hauerwas understands liberalism to be

> that impulse deriving from the Enlightenment project to free all people from the chains of their historical particularity in the name of freedom. As an epistemological position liberalism is the attempt to defend a foundationalism in order to free reason from being determined by any particularistic tradition. Politically liberalism makes the individual the supreme unit of society, thus making the political task the securing of cooperation between arbitrary units of desire. (1985a: 18)

A friendly critic might ask what difficulty lies in the practice of using the language of liberalism. After all, as long as Christian convictions are not distorted, what is the harm of framing the arguments for a broader public? The theological ethicist would have a wider audience and perhaps a wider influence.

Hauerwas answers clearly: the language of liberalism, insofar as it presents a coherent alternative to Christian convictions, is a language that is foreign to the commitments of the Christian community.[1] He is concerned here both with the substance of liberalism and with the problems of using liberalism as an approach to morality. For Hauerwas, a commitment to community should be part of the substance of Christian belief. But liberalism does not teach persons how to live in trustful community; rather, it encourages people to pursue their own interests without interfering with the rights of others (1986a: 24).

Liberalism as an approach to morality is flawed because it presupposes a universal morality. For Hauerwas, there are moralities only of particular communities; a universal morality is an illusion. Not just liberalism comes under attack here but many Christian approaches to morality as well. Thus, for example, Hauerwas rejects the Roman Catholic understanding of morality based on natural law morality, which assumes that human beings can by reason alone come to an understanding of their central moral obligations. In this view, Christianity adds motivation for fulfilling these obligations but does not add any particular substantial obligations.

Hauerwas finds this claim that Christian commitments function only as motivations for doing what all human beings should be doing anyway to be misguided. He states that Christians have a particular morality because they have distinctive commitments. God has made a covenant with them and leads them on an adventure, and this God also makes particular moral demands upon them.

In his focus on the problems of liberalism, Hauerwas borrows from Alasdair MacIntyre's critique of the morality of liberalism in MacIntyre's book *After Virtue* (1981). MacIntyre holds that persons today live in a morally fragmented world, that there is no coherent morality. MacIntyre points out, for example, that persons arguing against abortion use rights language and persons arguing for the option of an abortion use rights language. The first group speaks of the rights

---

1. Hauerwas is not convinced that the current circumstances of the church are worse than those of the past because of liberalism. The situation of the modern church is neither better nor worse in his view (1985a: 1).

of the fetus, and the second speaks of the rights of the pregnant woman. Even though both use the language of rights, they mean something different by that term.[2] MacIntyre suggests that we are using moral concepts that once had a home in larger cultural contexts but today exist apart from that context. With respect to abortion, the result is that many persons assume they have a coherent morality using rights language when in fact they have only fragments of what was once a more complete morality.

Another difficulty stems from the assumption that morality's task is to help people make choices. According to Hauerwas and MacIntyre, the purpose of morality is to instruct people about who they are and who they might become: morality should be focused not on decision making but upon character. Furthermore, given conflicting first principles, people still cannot decide what to do on the basis of a supposedly universalizable morality. Yet they continue to live with the illusion that a universal morality helps them decide.

Hauerwas appears to modify MacIntyre slightly. At times, he agrees with him that people today live in a morally fragmented world, a world that thinks that it has a coherent morality but in fact does not (1986b: 73). At other times, Hauerwas attacks this morality *as if it were a coherent one.* Then he goes on to maintain that this morality fails to do justice to the vision of the Christian community (1983: xxiii).

As fragmented, life in the context of liberalism has deleterious consequences. People are much less certain of their convictions; indeed, their convictions appear to them arbitrary, simply matters of choice. People know their own finitude and recognize that they are not the source of value. This uncertainty leads to the ever present possibility of violence because no way of settling moral arguments can be agreed upon. Eventually people become cynical, even about their own projects; nothing appears valuable enough to merit their commitment.

According to Hauerwas, people try to find a way out of this situation by calling for more and more freedom for the individual: individuals can thus decide for themselves how to live their own lives. Even this preoccupation with freedom, however, is for Hauerwas a form of self-deception. The freedom that liberal society encourages people to seek is a freedom from all commitments and ties that in one way or another

2. MacIntyre argues, for example, that the one group gets its concepts of rights from Locke, while the other uses concepts from Kant and Aquinas (1981: 7).

determine their being. Time after time, though, people discover that they are not as free as they imagine that they should be. Still, committed as they are to freedom, they resolve again to enhance their possibilities of freedom. Eventually this very search is destructive: they find freedom only in disowning their past and working toward ever greater freedom from commitments in the future. Hauerwas proposes instead that people can begin to understand freedom only by owning their past, even or perhaps especially those parts of it over which they had no control.

Hauerwas finds problematic one other tendency of modern thinkers. In their attempt to create a universal morality, they seek to ground morality not upon some contingent event, such as the history of the people of Israel, but in rationality itself. Such a foundation, they feel, would give them the confidence to make the decisions that human beings are required to make, decisions that involve their and others' suffering for their own moral projects. Only if they have a universal basis for morality do people think it can be legitimate to have others suffer for morality. Hauerwas rejects this position, believing such a universal basis for morality to be illusory.

In such a world, religion, insofar as it is a particular religion, can be thought of only as a private affair, something that might help someone with personal problems, but not something that might offer guidance about how a community should be shaped. In this country religion is useful only so long as it reinforces the belief that there is never any incompatibility between religious convictions and America. Most theological ethicists are unwilling to take a critical look at American society and to distinguish it clearly from the community of faith. The result is that one may never criticize the larger society from a religious perspective because doing so will be to mark one as a sectarian.

The consequences of this combination of views lead to the ironic situation in which religion can never be publicly commended *as true and as having something to say about how public life ought to be conducted.* It has only to do with one's private life, appearing to everyone else as one opinion among others.

II. The Importance of Story and Community

Hauerwas wishes to begin elsewhere. He proposes to do *Christian*, not universal, ethics and believes that one must start by understanding what

Christians mean by the claim that they are sinners (1983: 21). They further understand themselves not simply as sinners but as adventurers who will be sustained by the moral resources given to them by God. These convictions "take the form of a story, or perhaps better, a set of stories that constitute a tradition that in turn creates and forms a community" (1983: 21).

Probably no single feature of Hauerwas's work causes so much surprise as his emphasis upon stories or narratives. His intentions are quite straightforward. Contrary to those theologians who wish to start with doctrines, he insists that the narratives of God told first by the people of Israel and secondly by the church are the point, that doctrinal formulations are only secondary. Christians learn how to tell a story that includes them in God's life. To tell this story they must learn what it means to be creatures. Most important, they must come to understand their existence — indeed, all existence that we know — as a gift. They must learn to receive this gift, because no other response is appropriate (1983: 27). Hauerwas identifies three claims here: first, we are contingent; second, we are historical; and third, we recognize God's story in the life of Israel and the church. That story demands our transformation, and ethics, he proposes, is the study of that transformation.

> In this book [*The Peaceable Kingdom*] I contend that Christian convictions do not poetically soothe the anxieties of the contemporary self. Rather, they transform the self to true faith by creating a community that lives faithful to the one true God of the universe. When self and nature are thus put in right relation we perceive the truth of our existence. But because truth is unattainable without a corresponding transformation of self, "ethics," as the investigation of that transformation, does not follow after a prior systematic presentation of the Christian faith, but is at the *beginning* of Christian theological reflection. (1983: 16)

Hauerwas thinks that a central failing of human beings is the refusal to see themselves as sinners. The primary reason for this is that they deny that they are contingent, that is, that they are creatures. They wish to maintain that they are the creators of themselves, indeed, that they are something only insofar as they are self-creators. Yet seeing themselves as sinners makes it clear that what they need is not self-creation but transformation.

Hauerwas then delineates what it means to be historical. He wants Christians to recognize first that they are products of history, that things were done to them over which they had no control, and second that they can make that past their own by claiming it and putting it into a narrative that gives them a sense of self. Hauerwas wishes to discuss history and freedom together: freedom is not to be discovered in constantly stepping back from our commitments, nor is freedom correlated with awareness. Freedom is not in making choices but in identifying with choices (1983: 38).

But this is not all. Persons can be free only insofar as they are called out of preoccupation with themselves, and they gain this kind of freedom by telling God's story in a community. Because this community is central in rightly forming a person, it is essential that it be truthful. Among other things, this means that the community will have to live the story that their lives are not their own but God's. The Christian ethicist has the responsibility of assisting the community in the task of being truthful. That task is not an afterthought to theological reflection but a crucial part of it.

This responsibility of truthfulness constrains the Christian ethicist, because it requires that the ethicist attend first to the community and the story that it owns. Unlike a number of theologians, Hauerwas refuses to speculate on the "truly human" without attention to the Christian story. He fears that an ethic divorced from both the Christian community and the particulars of the Christian gospel will end by being a legitimation of the status quo.

The understanding of the particularity of Christian ethics is but one aspect of Hauerwas's claims about the relationship between the church and the world. One of his most persistent claims is that the church, when it is truthful, is distinct from the culture in which it finds itself. Only when it is itself can the church be of service to the world: its being itself offers the world another vision of how things might be (1970: 40).

Hauerwas wishes to avoid two temptations here. First, he resists the notion that the church is composed of persons who are better than their neighbors. Claims that the church is distinctive are not claims of superiority but claims about the radical nature of the gospel (1983: 110). Second, he opposes the temptation for Christians to see their morality as universal. If they do so, they will be tempted to use violence to enforce it. Hauerwas rejects both the claim to universality and the right to use violence that he thinks is correlative to it. Christians rightly affirm that God intends God's life for all of creation; this claim certainly has universal implications. Yet they recognize that this intention has not yet fully manifested itself, so they must begin where they are, in the midst of history, giving witness to what they believe and hoping that others will find the form of life attractive (1983: 62).

Christians must give primary witness to the person of Jesus, Jesus as he is presented in the Gospels. Hauerwas does not reject church doctrines about Jesus, but he gives priority to the scriptural texts. Moreover, he recognizes that the Jesus presented there is not the "historical" Jesus but Jesus as he was understood by those persons whose lives he had transformed. This, Hauerwas argues, is all that we have and all we can know.

In these texts one finds that Jesus does not call attention to himself but to the kingdom of God. Further, Jesus showed what was necessary to bring one's life into accord with the standards of that kingdom. Christians are called to be disciples, to orient their own lives according to Jesus' life. If they do this, then they will learn to be disciples. Discipleship will not be easy. At the very least, Christians will have to learn to forgive their enemies.

Hauerwas explains this imperative by placing Jesus against the background of the history of Israel, the background used by the writers of the Gospels. To the Israelites had been revealed God's prevenient and provident nature (1983: 77), and the Israelites then had to learn to walk in the way of God. This means not only going where God willed Israel to go but learning to love others as God loved them.

Against this background, for Hauerwas, what Jesus did becomes intelligible, especially his obedience to God's will. Christians too often focus on resurrection at this point and look past the cross. Hauerwas insists, however, that Christians should not have any illusions: they are asked to be ready to suffer for their convictions. They are called to take up a new form of life, which will bring them a new kind of power, the power of God that comes from responding to this invitation. In responding they free themselves of the powers that currently control their lives.

Jesus' announcement of the kingdom encompasses all these demands. Hauerwas stresses the eschatological nature of this announcement, that is, Jesus' pronouncing that the world as we know it will end. It will not continue forever. To understand this, we must come to see the world as a storyteller might, with a beginning, middle, and end. For some, this might be reason for anxiety, because their familiar world will be no more. But Jesus also announces the good news that God has made it possible to live peaceably in the world, without violence.

Hauerwas argues that the life of Jesus is normative for Christians, especially his attitude toward the "outsider" and toward authority. Although Jesus' teaching was quite close to that of the Pharisees, his views of the outsider and authority differed radically. For the Pharisees, the outsider was unclean and could be rejected; Jesus, on the contrary, not only associated with outsiders but took opportunities to welcome them into the community by celebrating with them. In this way, Christians are to display their belief that God rules the world, not death or evil (1986b: 132). Further, these celebrations can take place no matter who holds political power. God's rule has already begun and does not have to await a political revolution (1983: 86).

What are the other manifestations of this community? How should it be known? According to Hauerwas, the Christian community manifests a readiness to accept the forgiveness already given by God. Hauerwas, in a twist on the usual Christian rhetoric, talks not about giving to and forgiving another, but about receiving, from and accepting the other's forgiveness. He asks Christians to forgo those kinds of control that they can exercise in giving, forgiving, receiving, and being forgiven. What they must accept is their loss of control. Then they will be able to live as a people able to accept themselves, their sins, and their past, without feeling that they have to tell lies to themselves and others about who they are and what they wish to become. But they can do this only because they accept Jesus' resurrection as the sign that they should begin using the life of Jesus as a guide for their lives, rather than seeing his life in terms of their own world.

Hauerwas thus explicitly counters the individualistic understanding of the person that he finds in modern society. He counters with the church, which for him stands against not only this society but any political society. Unlike modern society, the church is formed by the conviction that God rules the world, and it bears witness to this fact. Part of this witness will involve nonviolence. For Hauerwas, violence is a sign that Christians do not in fact believe in the providence of God but wish to entrust themselves to their own powers. Instead, in this time between the times, Christians are called upon to witness to God's work in Jesus Christ.

Hauerwas is much misunderstood at this point. Some of his critics think he does not pay enough deference to the institutions of politics, that he has become a sectarian with no social ethic. His response is quite simple: the church is his social ethic (1986b: 1-2).

It is now that we can begin to see how different is Hauerwas's approach — instead of decision, character; instead of universality, particularity; instead of liberal society, the Christian community.

III. The Distinctive Commitments of Medicine

It might be asked of Hauerwas why a theologian with his convictions would write about medicine.[3] Although many theologians are interested in medicine because it presents opportunities to analyze individual difficult cases, Hauerwas wants to begin not with an individual case but with the character of the person. Thus his approach directs him away from what he calls "quandaries" that need resolution. Why, then, his interest?

There are a number of reasons. First, medicine is a practice not explicable solely upon liberal premises. For most people, physicians still have a kind of authority. Yet if people were consistent with their liberal premises, they would seek to deny that authority to the physician in the name of their autonomy. Thus it is possible to learn something from medicine about this larger issue of autonomy and interdependence.

Second, medicine is at the same time in danger of losing what makes it a distinctive practice. The language of liberalism has made great inroads into the self-understanding of medical practitioners (1986b: 4). The language of autonomy has been made part of the physician's claims, and now, in reaction to those claims, it has become part of the rhetoric of patients' rights movements, which criticize what is occurring in medicine.

Third, Hauerwas thinks that he is advancing a "natural theology" when he discusses medicine.[4] He believes that simply having medicine involves significant moral commitments on the part of society. For these

---

3. It is important to understand that when Hauerwas uses the term *medicine,* he means nursing as well as medicine. As I observe below, this usage causes him some difficulties, but I assume that his intent is to avoid the health care bureaucracy's term, *health care worker.*

4. Hauerwas made this comment during a discussion of his book *Suffering Presence* at the 1988 meeting of the Society of Christian Ethics (15-17 January 1988, Durham, North Carolina). The point was also noticed by Vance (1986: 12).

commitments to be sustained, a community of persons is needed to form the character of those who would enter the practice of medicine. To summarize: Hauerwas sees an opportunity now to say something to medicine, to ask it to live up to what is morally distinctive about it. In the process he takes the opportunity to deepen his critique of liberalism and its influence in this society.

Hauerwas has some reforming intentions in mind as well. Among other things, he wants to give another account of medicine than that offered currently. Hauerwas fears that medicine is coming to be seen as nothing more than a collection of skills that are morally neutral. When these skills are used badly, then the physician needs training in ethics — offered, of course, by more-than-willing ethicists. Instead, Hauerwas wants us to understand medicine as embodying certain commitments that are not morally neutral. These commitments are not recognized by many in religious or philosophical ethics. The result is that the practitioners in these disciplines do not understand the delicacy of the situation in which medicine finds itself when they offer to help medicine with ethical instruction. Unfortunately, medicine seems to be taking up this offer of help, with fatal results, Hauerwas believes, for the activities that medicine has embodied until now.

Hauerwas's method distinguishes him not only from his colleagues in philosophical and theological ethics but from those who argue that the knowledge of science stands at the basis of medicine and the physician's authority. When Hauerwas looks at our disjointed world anew to see which fragments from the past continue, he identifies one such fragment as the physician's commitment to treat the body (1974: 175). This commitment comes to us as a remnant from our Christian past, a fragment displaying the Christian belief in the fundamental goodness of the body. Insofar as this has stood as a counter against those who would glorify the mind over the body, that fragment is relevant for our age. It reminds us that concern with the body is part of medicine's way of serving human beings.

But that is not how the task of medicine is understood today. Hauerwas believes that those in medicine who have accepted the language of liberalism mistakenly see their primary task as the enhancement of patient autonomy. It may be that autonomy is all a patient has in a fragmented world, but that conclusion is ultimately unsatisfying. Hauerwas demands instead that medicine should recall its moral imperative to be present to those who are suffering.

Hauerwas asks the community of persons found in medicine to reflect on the question why we have a medicine at all. Persons cannot say that they practice medicine in order to avoid death, for this answer is inadequate. Not only is the avoidance of death foolish as a long-term goal, but it leads to those practices of a highly technological medicine in which patients are not permitted to die. Further, persons cannot, if they are Christians, say that they practice medicine in order to remove suffering, for that answer leads them to practices in which they have to destroy sufferers in order to remove suffering.

Hauerwas proposes instead that medicine is an example of a commitment that persons have to be present to one another when the other is suffering in the body. Cure is not promised, nor the relief of suffering. Presence to the other is all that is and can be promised. In some cases, the fact that I am present is the aid to the other (1986b: 63). Indeed, the reality of presence operates as a critique of the usual distinction between curing and caring. Presence sometimes cures. Hauerwas observes how remarkable it is that people are willing to be present to the sick because, as anyone who has spent any time with a sick person knows well, the sick are not easy to be with. The sick are the "outsiders" to the human community; they demand a great deal from people and appear to give nothing in return. Yet in fact, the sick teach the health care practitioner. They teach what it means to be ill and how one may learn to live with illness.

The sick entrust themselves to healers even though medicine, along with the rest of human life, is marked by tragedy. Tragedy occurs because medicine is fallible and because, inevitably, medicine will involve conflicts in values (1986b: 51). The physician may practice the best medicine on behalf of the patient, but the best medicine may not be good for a particular patient. Surgery may be indicated for my ailment, but if I am one of those people who unexpectedly react adversely to anesthesia, the best medicine has not been good for me. Second, physicians may simply be wrong about what is good for patients and, as a group, prescribe treatments that are deleterious. The history of medicine abounds with examples of once popular and now disproved therapies. Third, medicine will involve conflicts, sometimes of goods with goods and at other times evils with evils. The physician may have to choose between the good of the individual patient who needs treatment but will flee it if his or her disease becomes known and the good of society, which requires that this particular disease be reported to public health authorities.

We do not want to admit to ourselves that medicine involves tragedy. One of our responses is to try to maintain control by using lawsuits and other devices to eliminate or reduce uncertainty in our world. For Hauerwas, however, tragedies are unavoidable: persons will be harmed because of what health practitioners do. Those persons who would be patients must give up their illusions of control and prepare for a fallible medicine. However, a fallible medicine also presents complications to persons who would be health care practitioners.

Practices such as medicine that involve not only difficulties but tragedies need people who have been formed to carry on in the face of tragedy. Such people would be able to recognize even the suffering, difficult patient as someone who needed their presence; they would not see in every death defeat; they would be open to being taught by the patient. In the story that Hauerwas wishes us to join, the patient is not simply an object of charity, a person to whom one turns in order to exercise one's Christian virtues. The outsider is essential; the outsider is valuable. What we find is that the outsider is God's good gift to us for our salvation. The patient is essential and not simply the object of the ministrations of nurses and physicians.

The difficulty, of course, is that professionals tend to see themselves as the initiators and powerful ones in these relationships, and in their power they wish to ground their authority. They must understand instead that their authority comes from the moral skills they possess, not from their scientific knowledge or their willingness to serve the patient. Hauerwas insists that persons in medicine need to be constantly reminded that they receive as well as give in these relationships with patients. In order that this reminder be given, medicine needs an institution or community like the church (1985b: 54). Hauerwas is not here calling upon us to return to religious communities in order to sustain an appropriate medicine. What he does maintain is that medicine, if it is to remain true to itself, needs a wider community to sustain itself, and such a community seems unavailable to it in our age.

IV. Welcoming the Outsider: Christian Responsibilities to the Retarded Person and to the Fetus

As Hauerwas see it, nowhere are the differences between a truthful community and twentieth-century liberalism clearer than in the discussions of suffering, the retarded, and attitudes toward abortion. Let us take each of these in turn.

Hauerwas returns to the question of suffering a number of times in his work. He claims that liberalism has us see suffering wrongly. Liberals, as Hauerwas understands them, see suffering as something that always should be overcome. For example, the suffering patient whose pain cannot be relieved provides the paradigm for the consideration of active euthanasia. In short, it is the reality of suffering that causes the most anguish for the person schooled in liberalism, whether a theologian or not. In saying this, Hauerwas does not wish to minimize the real and terrible sufferings that some people undergo. He objects, however, to those who, in their zeal to relieve the suffering, consider the possibility of removing the sufferer from the scene. Although "solving" the problem of suffering for the survivors, because suffering is no longer present, this practice is not one Hauerwas wishes to encourage. Instead, he asks, why do we assume that we have to relieve all suffering? Is that medicine's distinctive task, or is there another?

Hauerwas maintains that, for Christians, suffering is a time to display their belief that God rules the world. Suffering and response to suffering can threaten that belief in at least two ways. First, if suffering has the last word in human affairs, then it is true that God does not rule the world. Second, if Christians respond to suffering under the assumption that *they* must do everything to relieve suffering, then they do not witness to the fact that there are goods beyond those of this world, goods not under our control (1974: 188).

What is it, then, that Christians must do with and for sufferers? They should alleviate the suffering, if that is possible. Beyond that, they should make themselves present to the sufferers so that sufferers know that they are still within the human community, that suffering does not make them "other" and thus outcasts. Even if sufferers wish to believe that about themselves — and when persons suffer, they tend to — the presence of someone can remind them that they are still members of the human community.

But suffering does not simply present difficulties for those who would be with sufferers. For some, suffering raises questions about the very meaning of the world. One of Hauerwas's most important discussions of suffering occurs when he reflects on the suffering and death of children. Here he also takes up his understanding of theodicy.

Hauerwas argues that modern people divide the world into evils

70

over which we can exercise control and evils that we cannot control. Sickness is an evil that we think we ought to be able to control. Indeed, we should be able to eliminate it. Given that we can eliminate it, we do not have to learn to live with it. But, claims Hauerwas, this is an illusion of Promethean proportions. As long as there are children, some of them will suffer and even die. Our task, then, should not be the illusory one of trying to eradicate the suffering of children but the formation of communities willing to be with them in their illness. What we tend to do instead is to seek "causes" for illness, and we are defeated in this search in the case of children. For example, children who have not lived a stressful life are diagnosed with heart disease. Children simply are ill, they suffer, and sometimes they die. We wish to turn away from this. Or in a desperate search for meaning, we try to fit that suffering into some larger purpose. Hauerwas suggests that it would be better if we did not try to force suffering into some cosmic purpose but recognize that it exists and try to minister to the suffering person (1990: 79-95).

Hauerwas's experiences working with the parents of retarded children over a number of years have given him occasion to reflect upon how this society views the retarded and how it chooses to deal with parents who suffer because their children are retarded. Hauerwas finds that persons in this society tend to make two mistakes in discussing retardation. First, they assume that retardation is a terrible evil. Hauerwas objects to this assumption as a theological and moral mistake: retarded people may be different from others and may have different needs, but their retardation should not be characterized as a terrible evil. Second, many assume that most retardation has a genetic basis and that the appropriate course is to eliminate retardation.

Hauerwas does not regard in an entirely positive light these campaigns to eliminate retardation. They disguise, he feels, an underlying belief that being retarded is an unacceptable way of being human. They betray this society's lack of the will and imagination to deal with persons who are classified as different from the rest of the society.

Those who wish to eliminate retardation may respond that in doing so, they would eliminate suffering. Hauerwas tries to show that the usual conceptions of suffering in this context are overly simple. He makes a distinction between suffering that simply happens to persons and suffering over which they have some control, suffering endured because of some purpose that they have. Christians, he states in *Suffering*

71

Presence, must learn how to be the "kind of people we ought to be so that certain forms of suffering are not denied, but accepted as part and parcel of our existence as moral agents" (1986b: 167). This does not mean that Christians have to look for suffering; in fact, they should avoid unnecessary suffering. At the same time, they should acknowledge the inevitability of suffering.

In Hauerwas's view, the campaign to eliminate retardation often disguises the unwillingness of people to have those unlike themselves among them, especially when the company of those persons causes difficulty. As long as the general society believes persons to be most themselves when they are free from all others, this society will continue to be uncomfortable in the company of the retarded. Hauerwas finds in this attitude a false sense of self; he argues that identity comes not from independence but from needs as well. The retarded make people uncomfortable because the need of the retarded is obvious, reminding all members of society of their own need (1986b: 169).

Concern for the retarded, worry that they may be discriminated against, fear that they will receive inadequate schooling can be either a goad to change the world or a motivation to eliminate the retarded person. The same might be said about approaches to a severely handicapped infant. Some justify nontreatment on the grounds that handicapped infants will suffer if they live. What is left unsaid is that persons often do not want to care for the handicapped and retarded.

It is most insidious that the very imagination that enables us to identify with others also leads us to see those others with *their* difficulties and *our* appreciation of those difficulties. It may well be that the retarded do not understand their condition as others do and thus their moral universe is different from that of others. Hauerwas encourages us to learn to accept that difference.

Hauerwas acknowledges that he has some theological claims to make here. The retarded are those persons in whom Christians recognize God. To understand this, Christians must give up their notions of a deity who is totally self-possessed and totally alone. To live out that understanding in the Christian community is the challenge that will involve clarity about what Christians think makes a person retarded. They may learn that it is the retarded person's dependence, which turns out to be only one of the many forms of dependence that humans display and wish to deny. Hauerwas calls into question the very idea of being retarded, moving us to ask not "How do we care for the retarded?"

but "What kind of a community ought we to be so that we can welcome the other?" (1986b: 179).

The community is also important for Hauerwas's discussion of abortion. Hauerwas insists on exploring just what abortion means and does this by asking what it means for people in a particular community, not by asking what it means for all persons. He argued quite early, in *Vision and Virtue* (1974), that it was not clear that everyone understood what an abortion was. It was hardly a neutral term, and yet it was being treated as such.

In his early work Hauerwas argued against those who, depending upon some spiritual principle of personhood, felt the fetus to be only "physical" and not a "person" (1974: 150-51). Our being is first of all physical; I am who I am in and through the body. But our obligation to take the body seriously, even the body of the fetus, does not deny the existence of circumstances in which the fetus might be forcibly expelled from the pregnant woman. Hauerwas focused on the agent's perspective in the decision. In doing so, he avoided maintaining either that all abortions are immoral or that abortion is trivial, simply a matter of a woman's choice in how she controls her body. Here Hauerwas wished to argue that abortion is a morally dubious practice within the Christian community, but that all actions that have the physical characteristics of abortions are not necessarily abortions in a moral sense (1974: 148).

In *A Community of Character* Hauerwas clarifies his position. Here he more carefully argues the religious reasons to reject abortion. Consistent with his method, he focuses not on a decision whether or not one should have an abortion in a particular situation but on Christians' understanding of who they are and how they must be transformed. According to Hauerwas, Christians ought to see themselves as persons who welcome the other, and the other includes the child. Thus they have to ask themselves what kind of persons they will have to become in order to welcome children into the world. The fetus is another form of the outcast that modern society is tempted to abandon. If Christians reject children and use abortion to carry out this rejection, then they join with that society. Again, this conclusion does not mean that all abortions are immoral. But it does establish a direction for persons, a direction that carries over from the question of abortion to a number of areas of contemporary concern (1981: 225-28).

V. Evaluation and Response

Hauerwas has offered a powerful critique and the outlines of a serious alternative to the predominant approaches to medical ethics. In the process of doing that, he has forced religious and secular thinkers alike to examine their own commitments.[5]

Hauerwas has pushed to the center of attention questions about the point and purpose of healing. Thinkers are forced to reflect not simply upon the very difficult problems that confront us in medicine today but upon the very assumptions that lead us to understand these matters as problems. In particular, Hauerwas asks the observer of Western technological medicine to reflect upon the significant moral commitments that sustain medicine, the content of those commitments, and the means by which those commitments may be continued in the future. Even if Hauerwas's approach is rejected, the character of the healer and of the community that sustains healers must be considered by any thinker who is serious about medicine.

Yet Hauerwas leaves us with a puzzle. As we have seen, his theological approach focuses upon the community — the particular community with its special commitments. This community is the Christian church in the rest of Hauerwas's work. When he turns to medicine, however, his perspective shifts. On the one hand, he discusses the significance of particular Christian commitments on such matters as abortion and technological medicine. He advises that the Christian community might have to practice an alternative kind of medicine if it is to be faithful to its commitments.

On the other hand, he argues that medicine needs a community very much like the church in order to sustain itself. If this is the case, then Hauerwas has, at least implicitly, a set of criteria for good communities. It would be helpful for him to articulate these, and, more important, to tell how he knows of them. In brief, assuming he is doing natural theology when he discusses medical ethics, and assuming that natural theology involves our knowledge of God apart from the revela-

---

5. There has not been space to discuss a number of important areas in Hauerwas's work. The issue of narratives and stories is important for an understanding of Hauerwas's theological method. Those wishing to pursue this topic could begin with "A Story-Formed Community: Reflections on *Watership Down*" (1981: 9-35) or "Aslan and the New Morality" (1974: 93-110).

tion of God in Jesus Christ, it would be helpful for Hauerwas to articulate his own view of how such a theology is possible, given his claim that theology calls for particularity and Christian theology calls for the particularity of Jesus. Hauerwas might be very helpful to us in our understanding of medicine, but he does not appear to be consistent when he claims to be doing natural theology and a theology based upon the revelation of God in Jesus Christ.[6]

He should also come to terms with the possibility that such a natural theology would lead to an alternative understanding of liberalism and its stepchild, patient autonomy. Autonomy might be understood as the bare minimum necessary to protect patients from healers who do not understand the limitations of their role and who have at their disposal all the machinery and organization of modern technological medicine. Such a "minimal ethic," as it has been called by moral theologian Allen Verhey, might be supported as just that, given that the possible alternatives in our world are not only Hauerwas's rightly formed community but the technological medicine he criticizes.

Thus far, churches seem to have ignored Hauerwas's clear call for an alternative to the medicine currently being practiced (see Hauerwas 1974: 181ff.). Just as the church could present a social ethic as an alternative to that of the larger society, such a medicine would be an alternative to the technological medicine offered to persons understood as medical consumers. Hauerwas wants care to be understood as presence. That, for him, is the appropriate alternative to the focus on technology in modern medicine. But at least two distinctive kinds of presence are found within healing today, and I suspect that both are necessary in healing rightly practiced. One is exemplified by the old-fashioned family physician who knew both who you were and who you wished to become. We are in danger of losing that presence in a highly specialized medicine where patient and physician meet as strangers. In my own view, it is the lack of such a presence that has led many to call for patient autonomy.

There is a second presence, however, when we are seriously ill — the continual bedside presence of a person such as the nurse. If there is a place where Hauerwas has lost an opportunity, it is in the use of language about medicine and nursing. He admits that much of what he

6. On this point, see Vance 1986: 12.

has learned about medicine he has learned from nurses,[7] that they carry out the activity of being present that is central to a medicine rightly practiced. Yet he persists in speaking of "medicine." If he wishes to insist that both physicians and nurses share in being present to patients but that nurses do this better in the current circumstances of health care, he should make this clear. I am not maintaining (nor, certainly, is Hauerwas) that these commitments are found distributed either by gender or by profession. I am simply noticing that the profession of nursing appears to embody these commitments to caring and presence at least as often as does the practice of medicine. Of course, there are significant counterexamples: nurses can be as oriented to cure through technological means as the most invasive of physicians, and some physicians are as committed to care understood as presence as the most compassionate nurse. It is simply surprising that Hauerwas has not more explicitly attended to where he has learned what he has learned and then attended to his language. Perhaps the categories of medicine and nursing should be replaced by the category of healing. If that were the case, Hauerwas might more easily enter into conversation with some Christian feminists. Of course, Hauerwas would find a feminism shaped by liberalism antithetical to many of his proposals. However, there are varieties of feminism whose representatives would be more sympathetic and yet challenging conversation partners.[8]

I offer these comments not with any claim that they point to fatal flaws in Hauerwas's project. They are offered in the hope that they will challenge Professor Hauerwas to think anew about the relationship between medicine and the church, between health and faith in this era of technological medicine. His contribution to that conversation has been both distinctive and distinguished, and one can only hope to hear more from him on these issues.

7. Hauerwas reported this in a conversation at the meeting of the Society of Christian Ethics, 15-17 January 1988, in Durham, North Carolina.

8. I have in mind here thinkers such as Watson (1989). Watson has some valuable things to say about the transformations of the healer and the patient that can be brought about by each other.

For one attempt to point to different forms of Christian feminism, and some of the implications of those differences, see Parsons (1991).

References

Hauerwas, Stanley. 1970. "Politics, Vision, and the Common Good." *Crosscurrents* 20, no. 3 (Fall): 399-414.

————. 1974. *Vision and Virtue.* Notre Dame, Ind.: Fides Publishers.

————. 1975. *Character and the Christian Life: A Study in Theological Ethics.* San Antonio, Tex.: Trinity University Press.

————. 1977. *Truthfulness and Tragedy.* Notre Dame, Ind.: University of Notre Dame Press.

————. 1981. *A Community of Character.* Notre Dame, Ind.: University of Notre Dame Press.

————. 1983. *The Peaceable Kingdom.* Notre Dame, Ind.: University of Notre Dame Press.

————. 1985a. *Against the Nations: War and Survival in a Liberal Society.* Minneapolis: Winston Press.

————. 1985b. "On Medicine and Virtue: A Response." In *Virtue and Medicine,* ed. Earl Shelp, 374-55. Dordrecht: D. Reidel.

————. 1985c. "Time and History in Theological Ethics: The Work of James Gustafson." *Journal of Religious Ethics* 13, no. 1 (Fall): 3-21.

————. 1986a. "How Christian Universities Contribute to the Corruption of Youth: Church and University in a Confused Age." *Katallagete* (Summer): 21-28.

————. 1986b. *Suffering Presence.* Notre Dame, Ind.: University of Notre Dame Press.

————. 1990. *Naming the Silences: God, Medicine, and the Problem of Suffering.* Grand Rapids, Mich.: Wm. B. Eerdmans Publishing Co.

MacIntyre, Alasdair. 1981. *After Virtue.* Notre Dame, Ind.: University of Notre Dame Press.

Parsons, Susan. 1991. "Feminist Reflections on Embodiment and Sexuality." *Studies in Christian Ethics* 4, no. 2: 16-28.

Vance, Richard P. 1986. "Medical Ethics in the Absence of a Consensus." *Books and Religion* 14, no. 10 (December): 5, 12.

Vanderpool, Harold Y. 1986. "The Wesleyan-Methodist Tradition." In *Caring and Curing: Health and Medicine in the Western Religious Traditions,* ed. Ronald L. Numbers and Darrel W. Amundsen, 317-53. New York: Macmillan.

Watson, Jean. 1989. "Human Caring and Suffering: A Subjective Model for Health Sciences." In *They Shall Not Hurt: Human Suffering and Human Caring,* ed. Rodney L. Taylor and Jean Watson, 125-35. Boulder: Colorado Associated University Press.

ON RICHARD McCORMICK

Reason and Faith in Post–Vatican II Catholic Ethics

LISA SOWLE CAHILL

RICHARD McCORMICK has long-standing credentials as a Roman Catholic moral theologian both within and outside his own church. From 1965 to 1987 he composed "Notes on Moral Theology" for the scholarly journal *Theological Studies*, covering and criticizing the international field; he has been a seminary and university professor for over four decades; he has also served on ethics committees of the American Hospital Association, Catholic Health Association, American Fertility Society, and National Hospice Association, on the Ethics Advisory Board of the Department of Health, Education and Welfare, and on the President's Commission on Bioethics. McCormick sees moral theology as a critical mediator between church and culture, bringing to the church a renewed foundation in human life and community, and to the culture a heightened sense of the dignity and worth of all persons, and of the right of all to participate in the common good. He is convinced that there are certain basic values to which all human persons and communities are sensitive, and that these can form the basis of public discourse and moral conversations among different religions and cultures. This is a typically Roman Catholic ("natural law") assumption. At the same time, he values the roles of scripture, religious ideals, and church guidance in highlighting and reinforcing human moral values and duties. The more specifically religious aspects of ethics have become more prominent in Catholic thought since the renewal movements of the 1960s, inspired by the Second Vatican Council.

Despite his Catholic identity and his commitment to shared moral discourse and to the revival of religious values, McCormick was once described by a conservative columnist — prone to hyperbole — as "one of the most dangerous men in America" (McCormick 1989: 6).[1] In personal correspondence, a fellow Jesuit addressed him, "Dear Enemy of the Holy Father." And this of the man whose motto and advice to younger moral theologians has been to maintain intellectual firmness in sure moral matters but liberty in disputed ones; and, in any event, to conduct oneself with charity, clarity, and moderation.[2] Those epithets reveal interesting things about the church context in which McCormick works, as well as about his own role as a moralist. Why have McCormick's critiques of Catholic morality, by cultural standards quite mild, been targeted by reactionary extremists within the church itself? And will his revisions have any impact on the moral theology of the future? How does McCormick's work itself both exhibit and enhance deep changes in the way contemporary Catholicism envisions its past, its contemporary cultural settings, and its message for individuals and for society?

This essay begins with a brief overview of the historical context of McCormick's work in moral theology, followed by a focused discussion of the relationship he finds between faith and ethics. (The relation between Christian identity and general human morality has been a special issue for Catholicism since the Second Vatican Council.) I then consider a topic that illustrates many of McCormick's concerns about the natural law method, Christian commitment, and the role of church teaching: the ethics of causing death either directly or indirectly, especially within a medical context.

---

1. The column quoted is Patrick Riley, "Fr. Richard McCormick: Theologian as Ethicist," *National Catholic Register,* the date of which McCormick believes to have been 1978.

2. "[A] simple counsel: *in certis firmitas, in dubiis libertas, in omnibus caritas.* And if one is permitted to expand the Augustinian axiom, *in obscuris claritas*" (McCormick 1984b: 138).

McCormick and the Roman Catholic Context

Since the 1960s, the method and substance of Catholic moral theology have undergone considerable reevaluation; the process has not always resulted in harmonious understanding within the church about its future. Some of the key questions are: Who or what defines the content of Catholic ethics and its relationship to "faith"? When is moral controversy within the church productive, and when is it destructive? More fundamentally, on what intellectual or theological bases is Catholic moral teaching grounded? Do Catholic moral teaching and the reasons given for it apply to Catholics only, or can this teaching seek a broader audience, make a wider intellectual appeal, and influence social policy? In bioethical issues like sterilization, reproductive technologies, abortion, and withdrawal of life-prolonging treatment, these questions have taken on particular urgency and an often inflammatory tone. In a volume that synthesizes much of his earlier work, *The Critical Calling: Reflections on Moral Dilemmas Since Vatican II* (1989), McCormick tackles not only some specific moral analyses but also the broader ecclesial context in which they are so heatedly debated.[3]

If McCormick were situated on a scale of Catholic theologians, he would fall into the category "moderately progressive" — loyal to Catholic tradition's essential values, but slightly left of center in relation to current official teaching. To be more specific, he disagrees with official teaching by accepting artificial birth control, artificial reproductive techniques when used between spouses, and abortion when the life of the mother is endangered; he questions whether the embryo can be regarded as a "person" in the preimplantation stages. He also argues that withdrawal of artificial nutrition and hydration can be accommodated under traditional Catholic teaching, which some other Catholic moral theologians (though not the *magisterium,* or the teaching authority of the Catholic church) have vehemently denied. He remains in the mainstream of Catholicism, however — and thus has probably more in common with his intra-ecclesial critics than he has against them — by affirming the value of unborn life and the weighty reasons against the

---

3. The need for moderation and good faith in dicussion within the Roman Catholic church is the major theme of the first half of this new volume. Sample chapters are "Moral Theology Since Vatican II: Clarity or Chaos?" "Dissent in the Church: Loyalty or Liability?" "L'Affaire Curran," and "Moral Theology Today: Is Pluralism Pathogenic?"

great majority of abortions; by envisioning permanent, heterosexual marriage as the normative context both for sex and for procreation; and by rejecting donor reproductive methods and direct killing of critically ill patients.[4]

McCormick has defended these positions by endorsing an approach that its detractors, including John Finnis (1983) and Germain Grisez (1983), call *proportionalism*. Put simply, this moral approach evaluates a moral decision by giving a good deal of attention to the proportion in the concrete act between its good and bad effects. Because this approach not infrequently results in challenges to the magisterium's definition of some acts as "intrinsically evil" no matter what the consequences (e.g., contraception), it has not received favorable reviews from traditionalist Catholic theologians or church authorities. To them, proportionalism is little more than a subjective utilitarianism that threatens to erode the very foundations of moral judgment. Revisionists, however, point out that genuine objectivity in ethics requires sensitivity to the *objective* individuality of moral dilemmas. Right and wrong in concrete cases are not always covered adequately by absolute moral rules which label certain acts — taken quite apart from any possibly mitigating circumstances — to be "sinful." Richard McCormick has greatly influenced revisionist thinking in the United States, especially by bringing into the conversation some of the more innovative Catholic authors in Europe.[5]

Revisionist controversies notwithstanding, McCormick remains true to a very basic commitment that underlies the Roman Catholic tradition of moral teaching: moral values and obligations are grounded

4. These positions are developed in many essays and articles. Most recently, reference is made to all in *The Critical Calling* (1989).

5. The discussion about proportionalism is rather technical, and it derives from the work of several authors (including Peter Knauer, Bruno Schüller, Josef Fuchs, and Louis Janssens) who have reexamined the foundations and functions of the "principle of double effect." A primary locus of McCormick's contributions has been his annual bibliographical essay in the March issue of *Theological Studies*, a scholarly journal sponsored by the Society of Jesus, and published by Georgetown University. See also McCormick and Ramsey 1978, which consists of McCormick's Pere Marquette Theology Lecture, *Ambiguity in Moral Choice* (also published in 1973a), the responses of several critics, and McCormick's response to them. Another resource that gives access to some Continental contributions is Curran and McCormick 1979. For a view of the general context of the debate and of more recent developments, see Hoose 1988. For negative reactions to the revisionist moves, see Finnis 1983 and Grisez 1983.

in a moral order known by human reason reflecting on experience. This commitment to an objective and reasonable morality is grounded in the thought of Thomas Aquinas, who in turn drew on Aristotle as well as on Christian sources. Although humans and their abilities are limited, it is at least in principle possible for them not only to become aware of those goods or values which enhance human life but also to consider these goods and values from the viewpoints of persons and groups different in culture, religion, or historical era. Human "nature" is, at least in its essential respects, everywhere the same. To know the moral law, therefore, is not directly dependent on faith or church teaching, nor limited to the Christian tradition. Faith provides confidence in the Creator of human nature, and motivation to obey the natural moral law, but that law is, at least in theory, a common law for humanity.

Since the 1960s, at least four important shifts in the Catholic understanding of natural law have shaken what appeared to be a prior unanimity of this tradition, both in foundations and in specific moral norms. First is a widely noted shift *from a "classicist" to a "historically conscious" worldview*. For instance, in the moral theology seminary manuals of one hundred years ago, human nature was conceived as a fairly static set of capacities and goals, of which reason yields not only unvarying but quite detailed knowledge. The natural moral law and the requirements of virtue could hence be formulated via a few basic principles and distinctions (e.g., double effect, totality, ordinary and extraordinary means). From these, all applications to cases supposedly could be deduced with a clarity and certainty that a practicing physician today might covet. McCormick has stated autobiographically, "Trained in the classicist mentality, I have become conscious of both its strengths and its weaknesses — and the need to correct or modify the latter" (1987: 37).

The twentieth century, with its development of the historical and human sciences, brought into Catholic consciousness a new awareness that an ethics based on "natural law" is, after all, fundamentally based on human experience. Moral reason reflecting on experience always does so within a historical context; hence its conclusions are to some degree partial and provisional even when carried out by ecclesial representatives. "Reason" in ethics stands for a quite complex mode of human apprehension of the good. As McCormick points out, "there are factors at work in moral convictions that are reasonable but not always reducible to the clear and distinct ideas that the term 'human reason'

82

can mistakenly suggest" (1989: 197). "Natural law" ethics seen from a more historically self-critical standpoint offers potential for a broad human community of moral discourse, but perhaps not absolute certitude about the transcultural and timeless adequacy of every specific conclusion, even those already proposed authoritatively as demands of the "natural moral law."

Second, the theological ferment after Vatican II has brought a greater awareness that the teaching office of the Catholic church *interprets natural law;* it does not simply transmit revelation. This has led to a problem. If natural law thinking depends on the reasonable interpretation of experience, and if the church interprets natural law, then is the church obligated to make reasonable and persuasive arguments on behalf of its teachings? What if its "natural law" conclusions do not appear persuasive to many either within or outside the Catholic church? Are those conclusions still authoritative? If so, on what grounds? Debate over these questions has led occasionally to polarization within Catholicism between those who advocate the tradition alone as the true bearer of moral teaching and those who believe the tradition itself must be accountable to human experience seen anew and so must permit significant moral reformulations.

Third, the Second Vatican Council represents an ecumenical movement toward dialogue with Protestant theology and ethics, and hence to an enhanced Catholic *appreciation for scripture.* Is a "natural law" ethics adequate as a Christian biblical ethics? Even if a "reasonable" approach to "common human experience" opens the door to inter-religious and cross-cultural concerns and to public policy involvement, does it do justice to the example and teaching of Jesus, with his radical demands for love and self-sacrifice? How can a Catholic ethics in anything like the traditional "natural law" form be fully a Christian ethics? In the Catholic tradition, moral conclusions have *not* usually been grounded explicitly in a faith perspective. What role, then, does faith play in the development of such conclusions?

Fourth, a more integral appreciation of the importance of the *sociality and interdependence of human persons* characterizes recent Catholic thought. Human interdependence, always a crucial part of Catholic teaching on social justice in economics and politics, has been recognized more clearly as an essential component of moral reflection across the range of morality. This has been true even in discussions of contraception, abortion, organ transplants, and use or refusal of life-sustaining treatments — issues traditionally analyzed more in individual terms. To base moral evaluation on the "nature of the person" means increasingly to look beyond the individual, and certainly beyond physical functions or capacities, placing the person in relationship to others. In some cases, broader social considerations have cast into doubt previously endorsed conclusions. Many Catholics (including McCormick) are raising the question of the consistency of the more flexible Catholic "social" ethical model, and the more firm "personal" ethical model of church teaching, used especially for sexual morality.

Some of McCormick's most alarmed critics are reacting in general to the incorporation into Catholic ethics of shifts like these. They focus on loyalty to past church teaching in areas of so-called personal ethics, particularly sex. A prime example, and for some a rallying point in defense of this teaching, is the 1968 encyclical of Paul VI, *Humanae vitae* (On Human Life). "Responsible parenthood" and birth regulation were upheld, but artificial means to these excluded. Traditionalist Catholics identify fidelity to the church with adherence to these conclusions, ruling out by virtue of church authority the possibility that certain past norms — in sexuality, protection of life, or medical care — might no longer capture and serve the moral values for whose sake they originally were formulated. The reasonableness of extant specific norms is not to be challenged nor the norms substantially revised. Loyalty in faith to Jesus and his Church is measured by fidelity to the Catholic church's authoritative moral interpretations. Hence the tremendous resistance within Catholicism — at least in its "official" or magisterial expressions — to "dissent" based upon reexamination of the original experiences or values upon which such teaching has been based. On the other hand, McCormick insists that the magisterium is not exempt from the ordinary processes of inquiry in ethics. Magisterial teaching must be accountable to generally available criteria of evidence, logic, and validity when it holds forth on moral matters (1989: 277, 281).

In this historical context, then, we can locate three main initiatives of Richard McCormick's work: (1) to develop the traditional natural law method into a more experience-based and flexible form; (2) to unite Christian commitment with the natural law method, which in the past tended not to stress any special duties of discipleship; and (3) to field issues of "dissent" in the church, making dissent a partner in the constructive development of Catholic ethics. McCormick notes that, historically, Catholicism has emphasized "the prerogatives of authority."

This makes it difficult to recognize "that Church teaching is a processive dialogue, not a once for all *ipse dixit*," and that "dissent, far from being viewed as a threat to authority, must be seen as an ordinary dimension of human learning and growth" (1987: 38).

Faith and Ethics

One asset of the natural law method in ethics is that it situates morality squarely in the context of basic human values and insights, thus enlarging the community of moral discourse to which Catholics can contribute along with persons of other religious and philosophical convictions. Christianity does not provide a "special" morality to members of the faith community. But does it or should it make a difference when natural law thinking is placed in a religious tradition, viewing humanity as created by and destined for union with God? That it has not made enough difference has been a basic criticism of natural law ethics by Protestant authors like Paul Ramsey (1951). By extension, this criticism applies to McCormick, and he has been sensitive to it.

In recent lectures, essays, and books, McCormick has become increasingly concerned to show what relation his natural law commitments bear to more specifically Christian ones. He asserts that religious commitment shapes one's perspectives, motivation, and process of reasoning in a general way and that it encourages certain insights. "Religious faith stamps one at a profound and not totally recoverable depth," and this "affects one's perspectives, analyses, judgments" (1989: 193). One's conclusions, however, will not be *substantively* different from those yielded by objective and reasonable but nonreligious analysis. "Christian emphases do not immediately yield moral norms and rules for decision-making," nor do they conduce to "concrete answers" unique to that tradition (1982: 29). As McCormick puts it in a volume on bioethics "in the Catholic tradition," Christian insights are "confirmatory rather than originating" (1984a: 59).

Among Catholic theologians, Richard McCormick has often been aligned with those, like Josef Fuchs (1983), who support an "autonomous ethics" rather than a "faith ethics."[6] In other words, basic human

---

6. For a thorough discussion see Vincent MacNamara (1985). McCormick discusses MacNamara's treatment in 1989: 194-95.

knowledge is possible independent of religious commitment. In trying to mediate this debate, and so include religious faith as an important element in even a natural law ethics, McCormick has found ethicist Norbert Rigali's distinction of levels of ethics helpful (1971). *Ethics* can be used with four meanings: (1) an "essential" ethics, which includes norms applicable to all persons; (2) an "existential" ethics, referring to the personal application or choice that the individual must make in his or her own life circumstances; (3) an "essential Christian" ethics, including moral demands made upon the Christian precisely as Christian, "which adds to the ordinary essential ethics of persons as members of the universal human community, the ethics of persons as members of the Church-community" (examples are regarding others as brothers and sisters in Christ, providing one's children a Christian education, and belonging to a community of worship); and (4) an "existential Christian ethics," embracing those ethical decisions that the Christian as individual must make, given his or her faith commitments and circumstances. Those identified with the "autonomous" school, with which McCormick is sympathetic, address the level of essential ethics, where explicit faith does not add "new content at the material or concrete level." However, "revelation and our personal faith do influence ethical decisions at the other three levels" (1989: 196). An unresolved problem here becomes apparent when one considers whether the Christian person still operates at four levels, or whether the Christian and human identity coalesce, so that there is one person, with an essential Christian/human identity and concrete moral obligations that arise existentially given his or her circumstances. In action, will the Christian person hold to ideals (at the essential level) that change behavior at the concrete level? This is the problem posed by more confessional and explicitly biblical ethicists like Stanley Hauerwas (1983).

Hauerwas would insist that to follow Jesus means to live a life that is demonstrably different from that of non-Christians. Nonviolence is the key to the uniqueness of the Christian moral life, but it can also be seen in stances like resistance to a cultural ethos of individualism or domination, support for children and the family, and willingness to care for the handicapped, elderly, or retarded. McCormick, as a representative of the natural law tradition, would not reject these ideals but would qualify them in two ways. First, McCormick maintains that the moral ideals of the Christian are shared by other reasonable people. Second, despite its strong biblical grounding, even the ideal of nonviolence is not an absolute moral norm to which exceptions can never be made. In a just war or in personal self-defense, even the Christian must interpret reasonably where the higher duty lies. Thus even killing might be justified in a conflict. A more biblically based author like Hauerwas would respond that the life of the disciple is a life of witness, however foolish the Christian stance of self-sacrifice for others might appear to outsiders. From this perspective, McCormick could be accused of not permitting Christian faith to transform "natural" morality extensively enough.

McCormick does claim that "the Christian story" has a fundamental and formative function in shaping moral vision. Among the "key elements" of that story, he lists faith in God as the author and preserver of life; the supernatural destiny of the person; the disclosure of God in Jesus Christ; the work of Jesus' life, death, and resurrection in transforming human persons; the guidance and inspiration of the Spirit in the journey toward full transformation; the identity of the people of faith as a eucharistic community and a pilgrim people, called to love one another in manifestation of the new life in Christ (1984a: 49).

The interaction of these elements with natural moral insights is elucidated in six themes of biomedical ethics that McCormick defends and elaborates in religious terms. Upon consideration, it is apparent that although the six can be expressed religiously, they are not all derived directly from theological affirmations, nor are they necessarily exclusive to Christianity. The six are as follows: the value of life as a basic but not absolute good; the inclusion of "nascent" life in the good of human life; the definition of the highest and only absolute good in human life as love of God and neighbor; the essential sociality of persons; the unity of the "spheres" of life giving and love making; and the normative value of heterosexual, permanent marriage (1984a: 51-57; see also 1985: 97). Christian commitment functions primarily to give a powerful backing to the importance of the six themes and their associated values, and to the motivation for realizing them in one's concrete opportunities for decision making. It is fair to say that virtually all of McCormick's moral principles and conclusions come down to a matter of "reasonableness"; but he increasingly uses Christian themes to flesh out and motivate. Basic human moral goods are known by reason, but the "human goods that define our flourishing" are "*subordinate* to" the "God relationship" (1984a: 37). In the end, then, he rejects a definition of Christian morality as a set of actions that the morally good pagan would not also perform.

However, he has tried increasingly to demonstrate that faith gives ethics an added dimension.

In a 1988 address to bioethicists, McCormick suggested that theology can relate to medical ethics in three "distinct but overlapping" ways. The first way is "protective." McCormick points out that while the moral agent perceives basic human values, the perception is shaped nonetheless by "our whole way of looking at the world" (1988: 18). In a technologically advanced culture, for instance, the Christian tradition can protect against a tendency to view persons functionally, by sensitizing the agent to a human dignity not contingent on social worth or function (1988: 19-20). The second way is "dispositive" (1988: 22). Christian faith disposes the moral agent to exhibit charity or self-gift in action. Citing Edmund Pellegrino, McCormick notes that charity can enter biomedical ethics (1) in the interpretation of beneficence, autonomy, and justice; (2) in the construal of the physician-patient relationship; and (3) in the way certain concrete choices are made. Although the concrete act chosen may be no different from that which a conscientious non-Christian might determine to be right, the act will be chosen and viewed by the Christian as "a more intense personal assimilation of the shape of the Christ-event" (1988: 25). The final way in which faith affects medicine is "directive." The biblical materials that occasion and ground faith yield themes or perspectives that "shape consciousness" (1988: 26). McCormick again lists the six themes cited above. In sum, he proposes that the contribution of theology to bioethics is "not a direct originating influence on concrete moral judgments" but a "compenetration" of faith and reason "to produce a distinct consciousness, a consciousness with identifiable cognitive dimensions or facets" (1988: 29).

A major objective of McCormick's recent writings on faith and ethics is to shift attention away from the principles and prescriptive norms that have occupied center stage in the Thomistic moral tradition. He focuses on the commitment of faith that is a response to the self-revelation of God in Christ. In so doing, McCormick follows the Catholic inclination to see Christianity as providing "motivation" for fulfilling universal moral commitments, but he does so in a more integrally biblical mode, tying his exposition more frequently to New Testament texts. McCormick's approach to the convergence of the Christian story and the human condition is particularly fruitful when he turns to the biblical materials themselves for insights. For example, he uses Paul's

Letter to the Romans (13:8-9; see also Galatians 5:14). In several places he makes use of the Protestant ethicist Roger Shinn's support of the continuity between Christian and wider human ethical awareness. Shinn appeals to the identity of the Logos made flesh in Christ with the Logos through which the world was created (1983b: 92; 1984a: 59; 1985: 98; 1989: 204). In interpreting love as the principle of the Christian moral life, McCormick forsakes any facile equation at the practical level of Christ's self-sacrifice with respect for natural dependence on and responsibility for others. Hence he corrects at least partly the Roman Catholic tendency to avoid recognizing special responsibilities for the Christian. Favorite sources are John's Gospel and the Pauline epistles (see, for example, 1984a: 51, 54, 56). Although McCormick reintroduces as well Thomas Aquinas's dictum that the form of the virtues is charity (1985: 104), he does so on the explicitly reestablished basis of a commitment to "love one's neighbor as Jesus loved us (John 13:33-35), even unto death (John 15:12-13)" (1985: 103). The meaning of gospel commitment for the natural law system consists in "a profound relativizing of basic human values." They are to be pursued in interpersonal life as the meaning of neighbor-love but are always to be envisioned as subordinate to Christ's love for us (1985: 106-8).

Yet, according to McCormick, the Catholic Christian's approach of "reason informed by faith" makes it "possible for the Christian to share fully in discussion in the public forum . . ." (1989: 204). He maintains that religious premises need not be brought explicitly into the discussion if this would hinder public discourse (1979: 156; 1983a: 124). Reason can be used to discover and debate the moral aspects of the human reality that the Christian story more fully discloses (1984a: 59; 1989: 203; 1983b: 92; 1982: 330; 1983a: 121). McCormick follows the Roman Catholic lead by rejecting views that a religious ethicist has no place in public policy, or that his or her function is simply to witness prophetically to religious ideals that will never gain a civil hearing. Instead, he argues that the Christian community has access to "a privileged articulation" of "common human experience" (1989: 204). It does not add material content but does highlight moral values in such a way that other persons of intelligence and good faith may respond. Religious commitment, then, does not "impose" a narrow morality on the public order but joins in a common, practical, and mutually critical discussion about which aspects of human moral obligation are appropriate matters for legislation, judged on the basis of criteria of common good and feasibility.

Valuing Life and Causing Death

New but expensive and often invasive technologies for administering medical care to critically ill patients have ensured that ethics in this area will continue to be of immense current interest for the general public as well as for medical professionals. The use of medical technology to delay death also raises important policy questions, as demonstrated by controversies over the federal "Baby Doe" regulations, over the ethics and legality of withdrawing tube feeding, and the advocacy of a growing minority who support direct euthanasia in order to avoid the technological spectre that the so-called new therapies can sometimes present.

Richard McCormick carries forward a long Roman Catholic tradition of reflection on the nature of the moral obligation to sustain dying or greatly impaired life. Current debates in the church center on whether the withdrawal of artificial feeding is consistent with the values preserved by this tradition, and McCormick's contribution to the debates demonstrates some of the methodological concerns that have occupied him throughout his career. Among these are the relevance of indirect and direct intention to the morality of an act; the usefulness of the principle of double effect as a way of specifying that relevance (evil results of good acts are permitted only as long as they are indirectly intended and caused); the viability of absolute norms specifying that certain acts (such as killing the innocent directly) are always and under any circumstances wrong; and the "proportionalist" argument that indirectness of intention may not be as important as the total configuration of good and bad effects that an act on balance realizes. McCormick has contributed to several facets of the discussion of death and dying over a number of years, notably on newborns and on artificial hydration and nutrition. Lately, his commentaries on socially costly life-prolonging alternatives have served as an excellent example of a social consciousness that existed in Roman Catholic medical ethics only in very muted form before Vatican II. Finally, in this general area of ethics McCormick has developed an explicitly Christian as well as a natural law perspective.

Ordinary and Extraordinary Means

The Catholic tradition has since the seventeenth century offered insight into the morality of life-and-death medical decisions by means of its distinction between ordinary and extraordinary means of life support.[7] In recent years, not only has advocacy of direct euthanasia grown stronger, but medical caregivers face new forms of the old "to treat or not to treat" dilemmas, in cases involving newborns or individuals dependent on artificial nutrition and hydration. A particular point of controversy has been the legitimacy of "quality of life" considerations in making decisions to allow death. McCormick's writings in these areas are fine examples of his ability to demonstrate both the suppleness and the commonsense basis of natural law thinking, while stretching it to new applications.

One of McCormick's most characteristic and helpful essays is "To Save or Let Die," which concerns treatment of critically impaired newborns (1974b). This rather brief and practice-oriented piece creatively connects with Catholic moral tradition, relating it both to religious commitment and to a reasonable hierarchy of values. Essentially, McCormick defends the moral legitimacy of withholding life-prolonging treatment from some infants and attempts to establish a general criterion for identifying them. That criterion is "relational potential." By relational potential is meant simply the "hope that the infant will, in relative comfort, be able to experience our caring and love" (1974b: 176). McCormick does not claim that this criterion admits of simple application. It requires determining that a minimally acceptable "quality of life" can be expected and making the determination on the basis of the child's own interests. It does not depreciate the value of the individual but affirms that genuine respect for the person demands attention to the prospects held out by continued life.

Central to the position is a view of biological life as a "relative" rather than an "absolute" value, one of the six reasonable but also religiously backed themes of bioethics discussed above. For instance,

> The fact that we are (in the Christian story) pilgrims, that Christ has overcome death and lives, that we will also live with Him, yields a general value judgment on the meaning and value of life as we now live it. It can be formulated as follows: life is a basic good but not an

---

7. See Gerald Kelly (1957: 129) for the classic statement. By "extraordinary means" are meant "all medicines, treatments, and operations, which cannot be obtained or used without excessive expense, pain, or other inconvenience, or which, if used, would not offer a reasonable hope of benefit."

absolute one. It is basic because it is the necessary source and condition of every human activity and of all society. It is not absolute because there are higher goods for which life can be sacrificed. (1989: 202)

This view continues the thrust of the traditional distinction between ordinary and extraordinary means of life support, which allowed that even readily available measures to sustain life could fall into the latter category and become nonobligatory when they caused "grave hardship." As McCormick puts it, use of extraordinary means would "distort and jeopardize" the individual's "grasp on the overall meaning of life" by submerging human relationships in the struggle for sheer survival (1974b: 175). McCormick discerns in this distinction of means the truth that life serves as the condition for other human goods and remains subservient to them. A keynote in his exposition is the assertion of Pope Pius XII that an obligation to use extraordinary means "would be too burdensome for most men and would render the attainment of the higher, more important good too difficult. Life, death, all temporal activities are in fact subordinated to spiritual ends" (1974b: 174).

McCormick identifies the good "higher" than human life as the capacity for relationships of love. This good is related to religious commitment because love of God is accomplished through love of neighbor, a claim made with particular force by contemporary Catholic neo-Thomists such as Karl Rahner and Josef Fuchs.[8] The derivative ethical principle is that "the meaning, substance, and consummation of life is found in human relationships, and the qualities of justice, respect, concern, compasssion, and support that surround them." If the physiological substrata of such relations are totally lacking, or if they are so minimal as to demand that the focus of one's existence be maintaining them rather than maintaining the interpersonal goods for which biological life is given, then life's quality makes its preservation not worthwhile to the individual. Life may be (not "must be") permitted to end by forgoing treatment. To return to the older terminology, the "extraordinary" or optional means must be defined in relation to the condition and prospects of each patient. An extraordinary means is one that offers

8. See, for example, Josef Fuchs's discussion of "Christian Existence and Love of Neighbor" (1983: 28-31), in which he draws explicitly on Rahner's essay "Reflections on the Unity of the Love of Neighbor and the Love of God" (1969: 231-49).

no benefit or offers it only at disproportionate cost, primarily to the patient. The commitment of the medical profession "to curing disease and preserving life . . . must be implemented within a healthy and realistic acknowledgment that we are mortal" (1989: 365). When physical existence is absolutized, it amounts to "medical idolatry" and often results conversely in abandonment of the patient when curing or even significant alleviation of disease is no longer a medical possibility. McCormick's advice to physicians is "Don't see death as the ultimate enemy" (1989: 365).

In more recent commentaries, McCormick has replied further to legal controversies over the physician's obligation to treat, or parents' prerogative to refrain from treating, abnormal newborns who are also retarded. Developing "To Save or Let Die," he expands the criterion of relational capacity into four guidelines extendable to other patient classes: (1) lifesaving interventions ought not be omitted because of burdens they impose on the family or others, who are owed assistance by larger social bodies; (2) even relatively significant retardation is not alone adequate reason for nontreatment; (3) life-sustaining interventions may be omitted in cases of excessive hardship for the patient, especially if combined with a poor prognosis; (4) they can be omitted if the anticipated life span is brief and if it requires artificial feeding (1984b: 121; Paris and McCormick 1983). As McCormick observes, such guidelines are an attempt to make concrete the relations of coalescent values and burdens, even if expressed in nonabsolute form. In this case, the rules "do not replace prudence" but are "simply attempts to provide some outlines of the areas in which prudence should operate" (1983b: 121).

This basic standard of worth of life to the patient faced with living it can function generally, guiding the cases of critically ill adults as well as of infants. The criterion in termination of treatment decisions should be "best interests," including some consideration of future quality of life. Following Edmund Pellegrino, McCormick has added some dimensions to the meaning of best interests, particularly for patients who were once competent (1984a: 115-16). The first component is "medical good," that is, a reasonable prognosis regarding the effects of medical intervention on a condition or disease process. The second is "patient preferences," based on the individual's life situation and value system, as previously indicated by the patient or as inferred by his or her proxy. The third is "the good of the human as human," a phrase referring to humanistic or philosophical values such as freedom, rationality, consciousness, and creativity. The last is "the good of last resort," the frame of reference that "gives life ultimate meaning." This will vary depending on a patient's religious and moral commitments and will affect perceptions of "best interests" at a fundamental level. Various religious traditions, for example, view differently the meaning of suffering or the value of preserving all life no matter what its condition. Thus persons will not always agree in their judgments of best interests. Nonetheless, McCormick as essentially a natural law thinker remains committed to the possibility of hammering out some consensus about best interests and quality of life.

This conviction is demonstrated in his attention to such court cases as *Quinlan, Fox, Saikewicz, Conroy, Herbert, Brophy,* and *Cruzan.* Quality-of-life evaluations will be necessary and not available directly on the basis of "objective" medical criteria (for McCormick's disagreement with Paul Ramsey's "medical indications policy," see McCormick 1978a). McCormick urges that decisions regarding incompetent patients be premised on their welfare reasonably construed; be undertaken by the family if possible; and be hindered neither by the confusion of treatment refusal with homicide, nor by the absence of some prior indication of the patient's own wishes (McCormick and Veatch 1980; McCormick 1981b: 107-10). The danger of "living will" legislation lies precisely in its tendency to create the impression that signed, legally binding statements are a necessary precondition of refusal of useless treatment (McCormick and Hellegers 1977).

Artificial Nutrition and Hydration

The question of withdrawing artificial nutrition and hydration is posed by the cases of Clarence Herbert, Paul Brophy, and Nancy Cruzan, all of whom were so sustained in a persistent vegetative state; and by that of Claire Conroy, similarly sustained and severely demented but not comatose. McCormick is sensitive to the belief of some (Daniel Callahan, with qualifications; Gilbert Meilaender; Mark Siegler and Alan J. Weisbard; cited in 1989: 377-78) that feeding by any method has great symbolic value. He cautions against its cessation, especially for incompetent patients. Nonetheless, it can be in the best interests of some patients to have artificial feeding withdrawn. Such cases would arise when the procedures are "futile"; when the patient cannot in any meaningful way be said to "benefit" (for instance, is in a persistent vegetative state); or when burdens outweigh benefit (1989: 385).

McCormick uses this discussion to address four central issues: the notion of a dying patient; the nature of artificial nutrition and hydration; the intention of death; and the burden-benefit calculus. A patient cannot be said to be "nonterminal" in any way that closes moral discussion about withdrawing artificial feeding simply because his or her life can be extended through the use of medical treatments. Some treatments may alleviate an underlying and otherwise fatal condition, but not all such treatments need be used. Transplants, artificial hearts, and dialysis all substitute for natural functions; but there is not the same moral obligation to use all these in all situations. McCormick finds that the so-called "difference between a dying and nondying patient" often "roots in a *value judgment* about whether we ought to use the available technology or not." He suggests that the appropriate value judgment depends on whether the treatment offers "a return to relatively normal health" and "ultimate independence from the technology" (1989: 379).

Further, he remains unconvinced that the nature of artificial feeding is not "medical treatment" and so is not subject to such criteria. Again, artificial nutrition is a technology that replaces a natural function. Moreover, death cannot be said to be the "direct" intention of withdrawal of artificial feeding, and so forbidden as "suicide" or "murder," any more than omission of other medical treatments refused by or for other critically ill patients. The moral evaluation depends on what a given treatment can be expected to do for a given patient.

The heart of the issue is the last consideration, the evaluation of benefits. McCormick disagrees that life in a persistent vegetative state should be construed as a benefit or value to the one in such a state. Instead, the interdependence between a person's biological condition and his or her ability to pursue life's goal of relationship must be considered. Demonstrating that it remains important to him to locate this basically philosophical analysis of the value of life squarely within the parameters of Roman Catholic thought, he concludes that "the abiding substance of the Church's teaching . . . is found in a basic value judgment about the meaning of life and death, one that refuses to absolutize either." "Those who would count mere vegetative life a patient-benefit have, I believe, slipped their grasp on the heart of Catholic tradition in this matter" (1989: 385).

McCormick criticizes the Cruzan decision, limited in applicability though it is to Missouri, because it seems to disallow any consideration of "quality of life" in allowing a decision when the patient has no clearly expressed prior wishes. "Paradoxically, in refusing to allow *any* quality-of-life dimension, the Supreme Court (with Missouri) is actually making precisely such a judgment. It is saying that preserving a life even *in that condition* represents a value to the person and a state interest" (1990: 11). Although he acknowledges that the quality-of-life criterion can be dangerous, McCormick insists that a policy favoring discontinuation of "treatment" should be developed, with appropriate safeguards.

> For several years, I have asked audience after audience if they would want artificial nutrition and hydration were they irreversibly unconscious. With virtual unanimity the answer has been no. These people were saying that they did not regard *continuing in that condition* a benefit to them. (1990: 12)

McCormick would also regard as morally acceptable the withdrawal of all artificial supports, for many of the same reasons, in cases like that of Claire Conroy, who was not in a persistent vegetative state. Forced feeding of the semiconscious elderly, often against their own efforts to remove tubes, can be dehumanizing. Yet McCormick also advises extreme caution in policy guidelines, lest the justifying "best interests" of the patient slide to social burden for others (1989: 386).

Mercy-Killing

Remaining consistent with Catholic tradition, McCormick has never defended direct euthanasia or mercy killing. Death in situations of critical illness may be brought about only indirectly by acts of omission. In an earlier article on death and dying, McCormick (referring to the work of Germain Grisez and John Finnis) locates life — at least that of the innocent — among the "basic values" that may never be sacrificed directly. He agrees that although occasionally good reasons may exist for omitting life-sustaining measures, the proposition that there is no proportionate reason for directly dispatching a terminal or dying patient has yet to be refuted (1973b). Weighing against direct euthanasia are the possible short- and long-term effects of accepting acts of commission. The "presumption of a common and universal danger" establishes at least a "virtually exceptionless" norm against it (1973b: 318-20). This is a social consideration that obviously moves beyond — though not necessarily making obsolete — the older Catholic approach that upholds the "individual's right to life" in any considerations of direct killing.

In more recent reflections, McCormick pushes again in the social direction, stressing the inevitability of human *interdependence,* so threatening to the Western view of the person as "autonomous individual." Demands for the right to control the time, place, and manner of one's own death, and the recoiling from any prospect of life or death in dependency on the care of others, require as a corrective the "incorporation of dependence as essential to our notion of human dignity." "As a passive virtue, dependence refers to the ability to receive other persons and their achievements into our lives" (1989: 218-19).

Direct Killing of the Innocent

Richard McCormick's concern with Catholic tradition as a tradition of reasonable moral analysis, his concern with its authoritative ecclesial expressions, and his willingness to be in dialogue with the hierarchy as well as with other theologians are drawn together in a commentary on a proposal of Cardinal Joseph Bernardin of Chicago. In several addresses since the 1983 publication of the U.S. Catholic bishops' pastoral letter on nuclear deterrence, *The Challenge of Peace: God's Promise and Our Response,* Bernardin, who chaired the drafting committee, has urged that an appropriate ideal under which to unite more traditional and more progressive Catholics is "a consistent ethic of life" (National Conference of Catholic Bishops 1983; Bernardin 1983, 1984a, 1984b).[9] The discussion of this ethic has ramifications for the discussion of causing death in the medical context, although its original primary targets were abortion (accepted by some Catholic liberals and denounced by conservatives) and nuclear war (accepted by some conservatives and denounced by liberals). A premise of Bernardin's proposal is that innocent life deserves protection, especially from direct attack; this includes fetuses and noncombatants. More broadly, the social question of the quality of life of all persons cannot be avoided if life is truly to be respected. Bernardin has also taken stands on adequate medical care for

9. Bernardin began to elaborate this theme in several major addresses in 1983-84 and has continued its development on several occasions.

the poor, housing, employment, education, and the cultivation of a supportive communal attitude toward life that extends to pregnant women and discourages the arms race.

McCormick does not quarrel with these broader concerns but takes up the question whether "no direct killing of the innocent" is an absolute moral rule. Here we see him probe more critically the position he once seemed to adopt with Grisez and Finnis, namely, that life is in all circumstances an inviolable good. Indeed, a more nuanced position on this point would be consistent with McCormick's own repeated insistence that while life is a basic good, it is not in fact absolute; hence, it may at least be *allowed* to terminate from causes external to the agent, if not precisely beyond his or her control. A further and more difficult question is implied if one grants that any nonabsolute good always stands to be outweighed, at least in the rare and extreme conflict case, by a good that is equal or higher (as in a situation of "life against life"). Could direct killing, even of the innocent, ever be justified? What exactly are the limits on the reasons for and means of causing death, and why are they so defined? The question regarding direct killing of the innocent can be organized in three categories: "(1) 'No direct killing of the innocent' as a principle. (2) The meaning and relevance of 'direct.' (3) The meaning of 'innocent'" (1989: 221).

In the first instance, McCormick argues that "the dictum [against killing the innocent] is a concrete rule teleologically narrowed to its present form, rather than a principle." The "stakes" in the argument McCormick is about to pursue have to do with the ostensible absoluteness of the rule. A general principle, precisely because it does not attempt to spell out all possible applications, may be regarded as holding in every case. It illumines a value that should guide the applications and the prima facie "exceptions." An example is the commandment "Thou shalt not kill." What holds universally here is the value of life and the prohibition of murder; what remain unspecified are the particular forms of killing that are to be counted as murder.

But McCormick notes that the prohibition of *direct* killing of *innocent* persons is much more narrow and specific, and that this narrowing has taken place historically on the basis of a weighing of those practices which do or do not favor the value of life in general. For instance, forbidding defense of the innocent against attack by aggressors would lead to widespread endangerment and devaluation of life. Any such sharpenings of general principles must be "similarly tested — and by the very measure or criterion that shaped the narrowing in the first place (the better protection and service of life itself)" (1989: 222). Rules derivative from principles are necessary and important but open to revision on the basis of the same value that the principle protects. "Such applications do not have the same stability, sweep and exceptionless character as more general principles" (1989: 222). The particular issue that McCormick has here in mind is the absolute prohibition of direct abortion, a prohibition included in Bernardin's "consistent ethic of life." McCormick would grant that the killing of a fetus is the killing of an innocent human life. Yet direct abortion to save the mother's life ("life against life") furthers respect for life itself, especially when without lethal intervention both will die.

Second is the problem of the precise meaning and the moral relevance of the term *direct* in delimiting the forbidden killing. *Indirect* killing of the innocent has traditionally been accepted in some instances, through appeal to the "principle of double effect."[10] Examples from the tradition include a lifesaving operation on the mother that has as an unavoidable side effect the death of her fetus, and the targeting of a military installation at which some few civilians are known to be present. Though the discussion is complicated, McCormick indicates finally that it is not always a simple matter to determine just why an effect sometimes counts as "direct," sometimes "indirect," if in neither case it is desired in itself (as in the direct killing or removal of a fetus to save the mother's life). Moreover, it is not clear just what moral difference the direct/indirect distinction makes, if life is sacrificed in a circumstance in which not to do so would amount to a virtual assault on the dignity of life itself (as in the old Catholic approach to a life-threatening pregnancy: "better two deaths than one murder"). McCormick's analysis makes ad hoc sense in relation to the rather rare prospect of maternal death in childbirth; it may have more troubling implications when brought around to the possible Trumanesque argument that not to obliterate a civilian population would amount to disrespect for life itself, given the alternate prospect of an even greater number of deaths in war.[11]

10. See n. 5 above.

11. McCormick himself has used the example of killing noncombatants in war — arguing against it — in order to explore questions and revisions regarding "double effect." Consult McCormick and Ramsey 1978, particularly McCormick's *Ambiguity in Moral Choice*.

Finally, we turn to the term *innocent*, which, McCormick observes, "may seem tighter than it actually is" (1989: 226). He suggests
reinterpreting the traditional stipulation that justly killed life not be
"innocent" to mean that justified killing can be undertaken only to
rectify a situation of injustice — but not that the injustice be the result
of evil intent on the part of the person killed. The tradition has been
inconsistent in allowing material injustice without evil intent as reason
sufficient to permit killing of an enemy soldier (who acts conscien-
tiously on behalf of his country); but not sufficient to allow destruction
of a life-threatening fetus.

Together, McCormick's reflections on the "consistent ethic of life"
point toward "the problematic character of translating the presumption
against taking human life into viable derivative applications for practice"
(1989: 234). In medicine as in war, the question is whether all norms
against direct killing are absolute, and if so, how that can be demonstrated. The rational or logical warrants for such absoluteness are not
clearly in place; authoritative church teaching alone is not a substitute
for such warrants once the validity of the natural law moral model is
accepted. McCormick's discussion is significant because it challenges
the tendency of much natural law analysis in the standard mode to give
more specific moral rules, dependent on historical experience for their
refinement and precise form, the same authority given to the more basic
values in which they are grounded, or given to the basic principles by
means of which the values are articulated and pointed in the direction
of practice. The discussion also demonstrates the continuing difficulty
revisionist thinkers face in developing clear and cogent alternatives to
the methods and categories of traditional moral theology, even though
the questions raised are crucial.

Broad Social Questions

In questions of death and dying, as in other biomedical concerns, the
social sensitivity of Catholic authors has become much more acute.
Through his involvement in policy-guiding bodies over two decades,
Richard McCormick has been a leader in reminding us that individual
treatment decisions cannot be excised easily from a social justice context.

His remarks on the artificial heart are illustrative. Although a
moral theologian of the last generation might have considered such a

technology using the distinctions between ordinary and extraordinary means, McCormick realizes that "an adequate discussion of the artificial heart plunges us deeply into social ethics" (1989: 260). Stopping short of comprehensive assessment, he at least challenges his audience with probing questions. Will this technology obscure more basic social needs? Will it "comfort the afflicted in their unspoken heterodoxy, 'If it can be fixed, why worry about the breakdown?'" Will it promote or undermine our efforts to deal societally with the elderly? What overall quality of life will the artificial heart enable? If the artificial heart becomes available, how will its economic accessibility affect our notions of justice and fairness? Does private financing of such options move medicine too far away from public scrutiny and control? "[W]hat is the impact of medicine's move to a business ethos on its self-concept, its practitioners, and its quality?" (1989: 260). The moral character of even a technology that promises to prolong life can no longer be resolved by a simple (and individualistic) appeal to the dignity and worth of every life, nor to an equally simple interpretation of the physician's duty to do the utmost for every patient. Research on the artificial heart represents a social commitment after which resources follow.

McCormick's series of questions demonstrates the need for interlocking Catholic social teaching — with its emphasis on the right of all to participate in the common good, the interdependency of rights and duties, the moral significance of social institutions, and the limited but important role of government in supporting the welfare and cooperation of groups within society — with the more traditionally person- and act-centered principles of medical ethics.

Conclusion

Among Richard McCormick's major contributions to medical ethics in his own tradition have been his dedication to the continuing viability of the well-honed terms and tools of the Catholic moral theologian's craft, and his commitment to greater inclusion of social and policy questions in moral theory.[12] His greatest contribution to the natural law

12. An outstanding example of McCormick's distinctively Roman Catholic approach to the sociality of persons in the medical context is his series of exchanges with the late Paul Ramsey over the morality of experimentation on children and other

method is to tie it more realistically to human experience and to individual and communal discretion, leading to the questions he has raised about the way absolute norms were in the past conceived. His distinctive position on the relation between faith and ethics affirms the ability of reason reflecting on experience to grasp essential moral obligations, but also much more self-consciously sets reasonable reflection within a life-perspective shaped by faith. He remains Catholic insofar as he stands firm on the common ground upholding diverse religious and moral outlooks; but he integrates moral theology with biblical imagery and religious ideals to carry through the impetus of Vatican II. Two critical questions perhaps remain, the first theological, the second philosophical. Can explicitly Christian and biblical moral exhortations be resolved into universal duties without actually being dissolved? Can universal moral values and duties still be credibly affirmed in the face of recent philosophical (postmodern) critiques of ahistorical and universal reason, and in the face of cultural pluralism? These questions set an agenda for McCormick's heirs, the Roman Catholic moral theologians of the next generation.

Above all, Richard McCormick's work is marked by restraint in the face of criticism and an unexcelled ability to sort through tangled Catholic quandaries of method and polemic, finally to arrive at incisive and programmatic digests of the issues at stake. His work sets a course and a tone that tomorrow's ethicists will find it easy to admire but difficult to match.

References

Bernardin, Joseph. 1983. "Toward a Consistent Ethic of Life." Address given at Fordham University, 6 December 1983. *Origins* 13 (1983-84): 491-94.

———. 1984a. "Enlarging the Dialogue on the Consistent Ethic of Life." Address given at St. Louis University, 11 March 1983. *Origins* 13 (1983-84): 705, 707-9.

———. 1984b. "Religion and Politics: The Future Agenda." Address given at

incompetents (McCormick 1974a, 1976, 1978c; Ramsey 1976, 1977). While Ramsey maintains that each person in his or her own inviolable dignity should be immune from "unconsented touching," McCormick argues that the sociality and interdependence of persons create a moral context supportive of proxy consent to involvement in experimentation for the sake of others, as long as it is of minimal or no risk to the subject for whom consent is given.

Georgetown University, 25 October 1984. *Origins* 13 (1983-84): 321-23, 328.

Childress, James, and Joanne Lynn. 1983. "Must Patients Always Be Given Food and Water?" *Hastings Center Report* 13 (1983): 17-21.

Curran, Charles E., and Richard A. McCormick, eds. 1979. *Readings in Moral Theology No. 1: Moral Norms and Catholic Tradition.* New York: Paulist.

Finnis, John. 1983. *Fundamentals of Ethics.* Washington, D.C.: Georgetown University Press.

Fuchs, Josef. 1983. *Personal Responsibility and Christian Morality.* Washington, D.C.: Georgetown University Press.

Grisez, Germain. 1983. *The Way of the Lord Jesus: A Summary of Catholic Moral Theology.* Vol. 1, *Christian Moral Principles.* Chicago: Franciscan Herald Press.

Hauerwas, Stanley. 1983. *The Peaceable Kingdom: A Primer of Christian Ethics.* Notre Dame, Ind.: University of Notre Dame Press.

Hoose, Bernard. 1988. *Proportionalism: The American Debate and its European Roots.* Washington, D.C.: Georgetown University Press.

Kelly, Gerald. 1957. *Medico-Moral Problems.* St. Louis: Catholic Hospital Association.

MacNamara, Vincent. 1985. *Faith and Ethics: Recent Roman Catholicism.* Washington, D.C.: Georgetown University Press.

McCormick, Richard A. 1973a. *Ambiguity in Moral Choice.* The Pere Marquette Theology Lecture. Milwaukee: Marquette University Theology Department.

———. 1973b. "The New Medicine and Morality." *Theology Digest* 21 (Winter): 308-21.

———. 1974a. "Proxy Consent in the Experimentation Situation." In *Love and Society: Essays in the Ethics of Paul Ramsey,* ed. James Johnson and David Smith, 209-27. Missoula, Mont.: American Academy of Religion and Scholars Press.

———. 1974b. "To Save or Let Die: The Dilemma of Modern Medicine." *Journal of the American Medical Association* 229 (8 July): 172-76. Also in *America* 131 (7 July 1974).

———. 1976. "Experimentation in Children: Sharing in Sociality — A Reply to Paul Ramsey." *Hastings Center Report* 6 (December): 41-43.

———. 1978a. "*Ethics at the Edges of Life,* by Paul Ramsey." *America* 138 (8 April): 288-89.

———. 1978b. "The Quality of Life, the Sanctity of Life." *Hastings Center Report* 8 (February): 30-36.

———. 1978c. "The Rights of the Voiceless." *Journal of Medicine and Philosophy* 3 (September): 211-21.

———. 1979. "Does Religious Faith Add to Ethical Perception?" In *Personal*

Values in Public Policy: Conversations on Government Decision-making, ed. John C. Haughey. New York: Paulist Press.

———. 1981a. *How Brave a New World? Dilemmas in Bioethics.* Garden City, N.Y.: Doubleday.

———. 1981b. "Notes on Moral Theology: 1980." *Theological Studies* 42 (March): 74-121.

———. 1982. "Theology and Biomedical Ethics." *Logos: Philosophic Issues in Christian Perspective* 3: 25-45. Also in *Église et Théologie* 13 (1982): 311-31.

———. 1983a. "Bioethics in the Public Forum." *Health and Society* (Milbank Memorial Fund Quarterly) 61, no. 1: 113-26.

———. 1983b. "Notes on Moral Theology: 1982." *Theological Studies* 44 (March): 71-122.

———. 1984a. *Health and Medicine in the Catholic Tradition: Tradition in Transition.* New York: Crossroad.

———. 1984b. "Notes on Moral Theology: 1983." *Theological Studies* 45 (March): 80-138.

———. 1985. "Theology and Bioethics: Christian Foundations." In *Theology and Bioethics: Exploring the Foundations and Frontiers,* ed. Earl E. Shelp, 95-113. Dordrecht: D. Reidel.

———. 1987. "Self-Assessment and Self-Indictment." *Religious Studies Review* 13 (January): 37-39.

———. 1988. "Theology and Bioethics." Paper presented at the Hastings Center, Briarcliff Manor, N.Y., 10 June.

———. 1989. *The Critical Calling: Reflections on Moral Dilemmas Since Vatican II.* Washington, D.C.: Georgetown University Press.

———. 1990. "Clear and Convincing Evidence: The Case of Nancy Cruzan." *Midwest Medical Ethics* 6 (Fall): 10-12.

McCormick, Richard A., and André Hellegers. 1977. "Legislation and the Living Will." *America* 136 (12 March): 210-13.

McCormick, Richard A., and Paul Ramsey, eds., 1978. *Doing Evil to Achieve Good: Moral Choice in Conflict Situations.* Chicago: Loyola University Press.

McCormick, Richard A., and Robert Veatch. 1980. "Preservation of Life." *Theological Studies* 41 (June): 390-96.

McCormick, Richard A., and Leroy F. Walters. 1975. "Fetal Research and Public Policy." *America* 135 (21 June): 473-76.

National Conference of Catholic Bishops. 1983. *The Challenge of Peace: God's Promise and Our Response.* Washington, D.C.: National Conference of Catholic Bishops.

Paris, John J., and Richard A. McCormick. 1983. "Saving Defective Infants: Options for Life or Death." *America* 148 (23 April): 313-17.

Paul VI. 1968. *Humanae vitae*. Boston: Daughters of St. Paul.

Rahner, Karl. 1969. *Theological Investigations VI*. London: Dartman, Longman and Todd.

Ramsey, Paul. 1951. *Basic Christian Ethics*. New York: Charles Scribner's Sons.

————. 1976. "The Enforcement of Morals: Nontherapeutic Research on Children — A Reply to Richard McCormick." *Hastings Center Report* 6 (August): 21-30.

————. 1977. "Children as Research Subjects: A Reply." *Hastings Center Report* 7 (April): 40-41.

Rigali, Norbert J. 1971. "On Christian Ethics." *Chicago Studies* 10 (Fall): 22-47.

Shinn, Roger. 1969. "Homosexuality: Christian Conviction and Inquiry." In *The Same Sex*, ed. Ralph W. Weltge, 43-54. Philadelphia: Pilgrim Press.

ON WILLIAM F. MAY

Corrected Vision for Medical Ethics

GILBERT MEILAENDER

IN OCTOBER 1986, on the occasion of its fifteenth anniversary, the *Hastings Center Report* published "How the *Report* Made a Difference: Reflections on a 15th Anniversary." Under that heading the journal solicited responses from six figures well known in the world of medical ethics. Each was asked to choose an article from the fifteen-year history of the *Report* — an article that had made a difference in his or her own thinking or in the development of the discipline of biomedical ethics. One respondent did not really select a single article, but of the five who did, two named pieces by William F. May[1] — the only person to have two of his articles so noted. Alexander Morgan Capron remembered May's "Attitudes Toward the Newly Dead," and described it as "a splendid illustration of the value of the humanities and social sciences for thinking about and formulating public policy" (Capron 1986: 9). Robert Veatch singled out May's "Code, Covenant, Contract, or Philanthropy" and suggested that it had "contributed significantly to [a] shift in public views about codes of ethics" (Veatch 1986: 14).

---

1. The unwary reader should be warned to distinguish the subject of this essay — William F. May — from two other men also active in the discipline of religious ethics: William E. May, at Catholic University of America, and William W. May, at the University of Southern California. William F. May held faculty positions at Smith College, Indiana University, and the Kennedy Institute of Ethics at Georgetown University. He is now Cary M. Maguire University Professor of Ethics at Southern Methodist University.

That May was the only author singled out twice should be no
surprise, for he is a master of the provocative, insightful essay — always
packaged in alluring prose of a sort one gets to read all too seldom.[2]
He has, however, written no summa. In two books — *The Physician's
Covenant* and, more recently, *The Patient's Ordeal* — he has drawn together and reworked views already developed in numerous essays. This
leaves anyone assigned to write on May's thought with the difficulty of
deciding how to package it. I have decided on a perhaps unconventional
approach. For the most part I will not discuss *The Physician's Covenant*
or *The Patient's Ordeal;* instead, I will return to the many essays in which
May first developed the themes reworked in those volumes. By means
of these scattered essays we may chart a way of entry into May's work
in bioethics. If it encourages readers to take up his two more accessible
volumes and encounter his work firsthand, it will have served a useful
purpose.

The Role of (Religious) Ethics

Perhaps the most obvious thing to be said about May's ethic is that it
is not principally oriented toward quandaries or hard cases. He is far
more interested in the images that shape our vision and thereby help
to determine what does or does not appear to be a hard case. He is
reluctant to adopt a single ethical theory — consequentialist, deontological, or virtue-centered. There are, to be sure, aspects of his view that
make consequentialism profoundly unacceptable, and he focuses a great
deal of attention on issues of character, but his approach cannot be
encompassed within any simple description of one of the standard
theories.

For May the task of ethics is to supply a kind of "corrective vision."
The purpose of ethics is to enlarge our vision, to help us see possibilities
that correct or transform the way issues have been considered. Ethics

2. Indeed, May suggests that our failure to encourage the essay is an indication
of certain (to his mind, regrettable) features of academia at present: "In a hierarchically
organized educational system, too much academic writing and speaking is essentially
filial rather than collegial. The two social vectors for writing are *up* (in the thesis, the
article, and the monograph), or *down* (in the textbook or the potboiler). Teachers have
lost contact with the earlier humanistic tradition of the essay, in which one attempts to
write *out* to an audience of intelligent inquirers" (1982a: 295).

as corrective vision "throws the world into a new light, . . . it opens up new possibilities for action" (1980b: 240). His focus is on those persistent problems in life that are less puzzles to be solved than mysteries to be explored: "the conflict between the generations, the intricacy of overtures between the sexes, the mystery of birth, the ordeal of fading powers and death" (1984a: 75). These persistent problems are best approached through image, symbol, and story. They "call for moral responses that resemble ritual more than technique. They require behavior that is deeply fitting, decorous, appropriate" (1984a: 74).

On occasion, May will describe the task of theology in precisely the same way: as offering a kind of corrective vision (1981: 133). He writes very self-consciously as a theologian, but as one who is present not chiefly in ecclesiastical institutions but in the modern university. In that context, he suggests, one cannot take faith for granted. But one *can* be certain that our world "reeks of religion" (1984b: 755). May does not mean by this that institutional Christianity is taking over our society. Nor is he thinking in sociological or functional terms of religion as a kind of social glue that holds a community together. He has, rather, been influenced by phenomenologists of religion, especially Gerardus van der Leeuw, who suggest that religion involves an experience of sacred power. In its different manifestations "the sacred is distinguished from ordinary profane power in that it does not appear as something that man can fully master and use toward his appointed ends. It confounds the efforts of the practical man to control it and the contemplative man to know it" (1972: 465). The experience of such sacred power and the yearning for it still mark our personal and communal lives. According to May, the academic theologian's task is to "clarify, interpret, and criticize those religious realities" (1984b: 755).

Thus, for example, when May characterizes death as a "sacral power," he considers what sort of "fitting, decorous, appropriate" manner we ought to adopt in speaking with the dying. Very often physicians, family members, and even ministers have practiced evasion cloaked in paternalistic beneficence. Against this approach others will argue that blunt talk, straightforward truth-telling is needed if we are to avoid paternalism, respect the dignity of the dying person, and retain authentic communication to the end. May argues, however, for a corrective vision that would open up other possibilities — in particular, the possibility of "indirect discourse" (1972: 485). Just as the ancient Israelites could not look directly on the face of God, so also death as a sacral power cannot simply be talked about straightforwardly. But it can be acknowledged and its anxieties confronted. The point is powerfully made in a passage like the following:

> My father brought this point home to me in the course of his last illness. At one point, he knew that he had cancer of the throat, but did not yet know that it had metastasized into the liver. In talking to me shortly after I had seen his doctor, he said to me, "Go easy, Bill." That remarkably compressed warning hardly served as an evasion of death. Why else would my father say, go easy, unless he knew that he was dying? Yet, he acknowledged his death in a form that signalled at the same time the distance he wanted to maintain between himself, me, and the event. He knew I had written in the field and he was saying, in effect, "Please spare me one of your seminar-length discussions of death. I don't need that now." I would have been a fool not to respect the boundaries he established.[3]

Story, image, ritual, and symbol are all central in May's writing. Consider, for example, one of his most influential essays, "Attitudes Toward the Newly Dead" (1973). In this one essay references to stories abound — ranging from mystery writer George Simenon's *Maigret and the Headless Corpse* to the story of Antigone in Sophocles' tragedy to Grimms' fairy tales to an Ingmar Bergman movie. May refers to myths traditional societies used to deal with death as Hider and Devourer. He gives many examples of ritual: phenomenological explanations of puberty rites, funeral practices in contemporary America but also in St. Augustine's time. And he refers as well to cardinal tenets of Christian faith — the resurrection of the body, the meaning of the Eucharist. All this is marshaled, channeled, and focused by May to help us think about the "problem" of organ transplants, the routine salvaging of organs, and related issues. It is hard to think of anyone else writing in bioethics today who could or would draw on a similar range of material to treat such a topic — and to treat it in a way that corrects our vision by seeing the issue not simply as a puzzle to be solved but as a human mystery to be explored.

3. I am quoting here from the earlier, unpublished manuscript of "Why Theology and Religious Studies Need Each Other" (1984b). May omitted these sentences from the published version of the essay and transmuted them out of the first person in *The Physician's Covenant* (1983b: 164).

If we want cut-and-dried answers we will, of course, sometimes have to turn elsewhere. There can be no doubt that we sometimes need such answers and that May's greatest strength does not lie in supplying them. Yet how thin they often seem in comparison to what he does supply! Thus, for example, May's treatment of organ donation and, in particular, the article "Attitudes Toward the Newly Dead" was targeted by Joel Feinberg as an example of the kind of thinking that — relying as it does on image, symbol, and story — falls into "the moral traps of sentimentality and squeamishness" (Feinberg 1985: 31). May approaches the question of organ donation, Feinberg writes, "more in the manner of literary critics debating the appropriateness of symbols than as [a moralist]" (1985: 34). May himself has responded to these charges and, I think, gotten the better of the exchange (1985b). He argues that there is not available to us what Feinberg seems to think we should use: some form of "symbol-free" access to the world. To imagine we have one is simply to fall captive to one symbol-laden way of thinking about a reality like a dead body (1985b: 38). Moreover, symbols and rituals help to discipline and shape our sentiments. To pay attention to them is not to wallow in sentimentality; it is to recognize that more than our rational powers will be needed if we are to shape, form, and re-form the sentiments central to human existence (1985b: 40).

May's style of ethics will not do everything that is needed, nor does he imagine that it will. Indeed, in the hands of a less virtuoso performer, it might be open to some of the charges Feinberg brings. But May is a virtuoso, and he has adopted a style that makes possible a theological ethic that addresses fundamental questions without denying whatever human insight can be found. He draws on as many sources of wisdom as he can — while never failing to provide the corrective re-envisioning that his theology makes possible and that, he judges, it is the task of ethics to provide.

Death as Sacral Power

One of the persistent problems that has occupied May's attention for decades and to which he has applied the method already described is the human struggle with fading powers and, finally, death. Indeed, May's never published dissertation was titled "Dread Before Death and Revolt Against Death: A Study of Heidegger and Camus." We are not surprised,

110

then, to note that May has discerned in our culture a twofold response to death: preoccupation and obsession, and concealment and avoidance (1972: 469). In his discussions of death we see, I think, the most fundamental theological influences on May's work.

Clearly he has been influenced by the concerns of existentialist philosophers Martin Heidegger and Albert Camus. Certainly the work of a phenomenologist such as Van der Leeuw has left its mark. But the most basic influence, I venture to suggest, is one rarely mentioned in May's writing. Perhaps I am mistaken; certainly one cannot prove this by quotation from May's essays. But the influence of theologian Karl Barth seems to have deeply marked almost everything May has to say about suffering and death. For it is the triumph of grace over all opposing, negative powers — a triumph strongly emphasized by Barth — that sounds clearly in May's work.

Of all the negative powers humans face, death is the most terrifying. In our time it appears as the great individualizer. In medieval times it was the great leveler. In both cases an alienating force. For us, living in an age of conformity, death serves to pull us out of the mass and make us confront our destiny as single individuals. For the medieval man or woman, living in a more hierarchically structured world, death brought all to the same shared end. In either case, the dying person came to see his culture as though a stranger to it (1972: 475ff.).

But the significance of death cuts still more deeply into our identity. May writes that death involves a threefold crisis. It is, first, a crisis of the flesh. The body serves as our means to control the world, and death threatens us with loss of control. The body serves as our means to savor the world's splendor, and death threatens a final loss of taste. The body is, most centrally, revelatory of the self, since we are our bodies. And death threatens the loss of self.

Those who enter the healing professions would do well to remember this crisis of the flesh and learn from it. If death threatens the loss of control, they need to provide ways for patients to participate in treatment decisions as much as possible. If death threatens our ability to savor the world, the healing professions must be alert to all opportunities for patients to continue to experience the world's beauty (including a concern for the grounds of hospitals or nursing homes). If death threatens the loss of self, would-be healers must think not simply of curing but of caring that extends to the smallest details (1972: 480ff.).

But death is not only a crisis of the flesh. It is, second, a crisis of

111

community. It means abandonment, the loss of communication. It calls upon us, therefore, to find ways to remain "in touch," ways that will usually involve the "indirect discourse" of which we have spoken above. Death will also reveal — starkly and unmistakably — something about the communities in which the dying person lives. It will reveal whether they are able to care even when they can no longer cure. Death is "that occasion in which the community, wholly divested of messianic pretension, is revealed in its humanity as a network of care" (1972: 488).

Death brings yet a third crisis — of separation not just from the body and community, but from God (1969: 181). Death threatens our self-integration and threatens us with "dispossession." This terminology suggests, however, that we need to think of the self within a transcendent context — as ecstatic, "pitched out beyond itself toward that in which it finds its meaning" (1985a: 260). The self cannot be whole in itself; that way lies only a final dispossession. The Christian gospel is addressed precisely to such an analysis, announcing that death's powerlessness over against the love of God has been revealed and enacted in Jesus. This frees us from the power of death as a sacral reality, frees us from either preoccupation with or avoidance of death. As May writes,

> To preach about death is absolutely essential if Christians are to preach with joy. Otherwise they speak with the profound melancholy of men who have separated the church from the graveyard. They make the practical assumption that there are two Lords. . . . The Christian faith, however, does not speak of two parallel Lords. The Lord of the Church is not ruler of a surface kingdom. His dominion is nothing if it does not go at least six feet deep. (1969: 176f.)

Here is the Barthian note that runs through May's theology. No ultimate dualisms are permitted. No other sacral powers can ultimately challenge the hegemony of the Father of Jesus Christ.

The dangers in this sort of view are well known to theologians and obvious to anyone who thinks about such matters. Such a view risks a Pollyannaish approach to evil, never really opening itself fully to its terrible reality. Since May tends to trace evils to "sacral powers" more than to human sin and then to depict these powers as exposed in their impotence by Christ, he regularly runs such risks. He also recognizes, however, that "suffering does not inevitably ennoble. Heavy responsibilities crush as well as enlarge their bearers" (1983a: 153). What May needs — and, at least sometimes, finds — is language that permits him to take seriously the evils of suffering and death, yet without elevating them to the level of the one ultimate power that has been revealed in Jesus Christ as wholly good and loving. The language he finds is grounded in the New Testament and, in particular, in the eighth chapter of Romans. Here aging, suffering, and dying are seen as destructive forces — "real" but not "ultimate" (1985a: 261-62). They are not to be denied or avoided, but they are to be treated with a certain nonchalance.

Nonchalance is, in fact, a central category in May's thought. It is a metaphysical nonchalance, made possible by the conviction that there is only one Lord and that his kingdom goes at least six feet deep. This is a major part of the "corrective vision" that theology supplies to medical ethics. We take suffering *too* seriously when we see it as an overmastering, ultimate power.

This point emerges wonderfully in May's interpretation of Fyodor Dostoevsky's Grand Inquisitor. The Inquisitor of *The Brothers Karamazov* is, according to May, a deeply religious man who believes in the ultimate triumph of suffering and the grave. But he is also an arch-humanist. Loving human beings as he does, he must do whatever he can to protect them (1972: 22).

Like the Grand Inquisitor, we often become arch-humanists, especially, for example, in caring for our children. Because we love them, we wish to protect them from suffering. "As conscientious parents, [we] operate as though the powers that are decisive in the universe could not possibly do anything in and through the suffering of [our] children" (1974: 21). We are forced to become savior figures, even though we thereby live a lie. We are forced, in terms of moral theory, to a consequentialism willing to adopt any means that offers relief of suffering.

We need to know that there is only one Lord if we are to stop bending the knee to the sacral powers of suffering and death. We need the metaphysical nonchalance that flows from this conviction — or so May thinks. If we know that these other powers are real but not ultimate, our attitudes and actions will be affected by that knowledge. "In allowing the self to sit loose to the world, it makes it easier for the self to meet its obligations within it, without panicking before it or getting mired in it" (1985a: 262).

This is, I think, the essence of "corrective vision" — and it is, as I have noted, central in May's work. In a very different context we can see the same approach at work. May suggests more than once that we treat death (with preoccupation and avoidance) the way Victorians treated sex. In the sexual sphere, too, we need a certain nonchalance. Only if we know that sexual pleasure is a real though not ultimate good for humans will we cease asking the impossible from our partner, cease hoping that the sexual bond might itself be salvific. Only then will we be free to enjoy the pleasure for what it is (1988: 39).

May has described this nonchalance as "metaphysical optimism" (1976: 223). Beginning from the assumption that the evils and negativities of life are not ultimate, one does not have to seek their elimination as necessary to a truly human existence. There is no need for preoccupation with death; only God is worthy of worship. Nor is there need to avoid or conceal death; its ultimate powerlessness has been exposed. We need not seek to protect our loved ones from all suffering; we are free to acknowledge the reality of their dying and ours. We are enabled, perhaps, to think of better ways to care for the dying than hiding them away in institutions designed for such purposes.

But in all this we should not fail to recognize the genuinely painful reality of aging, suffering, and death. Metaphysical optimism and nonchalance correct our vision, set us free to provide care. They do not evade reality. They do not translate into "gabby bluntness" when faced with the sacral power of death (1972: 485). But in correcting our vision, they shape attitudes and actions in ways that cannot be reduced to any formula yet can be seen to be "fitting, decorous, appropriate."

A Covenanted Profession

All human beings face a common destiny in death. All are, wittingly or unwittingly, subject to a still greater Lord who has taken the sting from death. These truths are of special importance for the medical profession, but we can begin with their application elsewhere. Karl Barth devoted the better part of a volume of his *Church Dogmatics* to characterizing "creation as the external basis of the covenant," and "covenant as the internal basis of creation" (Barth 1958). By this Barth meant at least to suggest that the created world provides a backdrop that makes possible ties between human beings. It sets the context for their coming together to share a common life and to come to terms with the reality of the other person. Human beings may do this in different ways, but it is (Barth also meant to say) covenant that is the internal goal, the meaning and purpose toward which our lives are ordered. To take up our relationships with each other and consciously to accept them as covenant bonds calling for faithfulness is the point of our creation as human beings.[4]

There is, of course, more than one way to structure a bond of one human life with another. The emphasis on covenant, so central in May's writing, can sometimes produce a kind of anti-individualism that criticizes any sign of adversarialism or self-seeking. In so doing it can nullify Barth's first formula: that the created world of individuals is the external basis of covenant and should not simply be absorbed or obliterated within any common life we shape. If the covenant is ultimately with God, we must recognize as May does (though perhaps not often enough) "the 'principle of extra-territoriality' in the relations of the person to the social order" (1973: 7). Human beings are not simply cogs in the social machine or parts of any communal whole. They are individuals whose lives are bound together in countless different ways. Their moral task is to take up these bonds, accept them, and shape them in accord with covenant fidelity.

Consider, for example, a retarded child and his parents. Since, seen in transcendent context, there is no such thing as an autonomous or self-sufficient individual, the child's parents cannot ground his "value" solely in any personal properties or capacities. The child always exists in relation to God, and his value cannot be derived wholly from care the parents do or do not provide (1983a: 159). The parents, in turn, simply find their lives bound to this child. What are they to make, morally, of the bond? They may adhere to a moral code that confers upon this child, as upon all humans, certain rights. If so, they will no doubt believe that they have at least certain minimal obligations toward the child. They will, at the very least, need to find a home for the child in one of those institutions philanthropically provided for such purposes (1983a: 157). If they do more than this, if they give their own time and energy to caring for the child, they may think of their action as philanthropic and gratuitous — more than can be called obligation.

But it is also possible that they may think otherwise. Knowing themselves always to be gifted by that one Lord who rules all, knowing

---

4. The use of this Barthian theme in medical ethics can probably be traced to the preface of Paul Ramsey's *Patient as Person* (1970: xi-xiv). This essay is, I suspect, another important influence on May.

themselves to be indebted in this way, they may take up their bond with this child and see it as one calling for loyalty on their part. Theirs is not a wholly gratuitous altruism, but a response to the fact that their own lives have been divinely graced. They will see themselves as indebted, not just as self-sufficient givers of care. And out of such a corrected vision there may even come a new mutuality in relation to their child. Their care will no longer seem heroic, for they may come to think that this child nourishes them even as they nourish him. "That sustenance [from child to parents] may be difficult to acknowledge without sounding as though one is justifying the existence of mental retardation. Yet some parents have acknowledged the deepening of their lives; they find themselves in retrospect a little kinder, a little gentler, a little more sensitive to the difficulties others face than they might otherwise have been" (1983a: 156). They simply found themselves thrown into a particular bond — the external backdrop for the moral tasks they take up. But they have discerned the internal meaning of this given bond to be covenant loyalty, a loyalty grounded in their realization that they are themselves indebted, that they are not self-sufficient caregivers. They have given more than the minimal care they owed — that is to say, the element of the gratuitous has touched this bond. But they have not thought of themselves as simple altruists but, instead, as responsive and indebted receivers of gifts.

Something like this is also May's image of what the medical profession might be and, indeed, is at its best. To call medicine a profession is to focus on the fact that its practitioners "profess" something. They profess, first, technical competence based on a tradition of learning that is university based. Second, they profess a moral responsibility to use this knowledge in service of human need (1980b: 205). To these must be added a third feature essential to any profession: an organized structure that makes possible professional discipline. "The natural form of organization that should obtain amongst professionals is collegial rather than hierarchical or competitive. The principle of collegiality follows from the insistence that the professional must have direct access to first principles" (1986b: 22).

Our cultural circumstances, however, make some of these features of "profession" difficult. Institutional structures in our society are hierarchically ordered. When professionals, whose natural mode of relation is collegial, work within such structures, they face certain tensions. As professionals they are equal colleagues; as members of a bureaucracy

116

they may be super- and subordinates (1980b: 223). The university basis for professional training has also become problematic. May discerns a fine irony in the fact that just at the moment in history when professions turned to universities for training, those universities were claiming that moral reflection and nurture were not part of their mission (1986b: 22). One's pursuit of professional knowledge would be not so much the enactment of a moral responsibility but a means to private self-fulfillment. Hence the professional's knowledge came to be viewed as a private possession to be used for personal advantage rather than as a public trust. The professional, in short, learned to think of himself less as beneficiary and more as philanthropist (1982a: 291).

What is needed, May thinks, is the sense of medicine as a covenanted profession. He pits against each other a code-morality and a covenant-morality. He does so not because he thinks code-morality is simply a bad thing. On the contrary, a moral code rooted in universal categories that govern professional performance is likely to encourage the development of technical competence. But it may also lead to a certain moral minimalism, a sense that anything beyond the minimum care for patients is gratuitous. May therefore corrects code with philanthropy, "an ethic of love without ties" (1982b: 35). By contrast, he connects covenant with a sense of indebtedness. Doctors have traditionally thought of themselves as indebted to each other — to the profession in which they have been nourished. They have, however, been less likely to think of their bond to patients in such terms. In that context they are less likely to think of their actions as response to gifts received (1975: 31).

Surely this is an accurate depiction of the attitude only of some medical professionals, but as a depiction it is vintage May. He contrasts the novels of Ernest Hemingway, which exhibit an understanding of life according to code, with the novels of William Faulkner, which illustrate covenant indebtedness. The Hemingway hero is epitomized by powerful technical performance — as, for example, in the killing of a bull. The classic performance completed, one moves on. Faulkner, by contrast, depicts the interior life of a boy who comes of age in a hunt, "ritually" slaying a deer and marking his face "forever" with the blood. "The Hemingway hero slays his bull and then it is over; but young Isaac McCaslin binds the whole of his future in the instant" (1975:31).

A covenanted physician is likewise marked "forever" by the claims of his profession. He knows himself to be greatly indebted to his patients and his community for the skill and art he possesses. He is not, in truth, a self-sufficient giver, and his morality cannot be one of universal categories alone. Covenants have their root in particular historical circumstances: the training of the physician in institutions supported by the community, the willingness of patients to hand themselves over even to inexperienced physicians for care, and decades of subjects who have consented to research.

One might well ask, however, whether there are not other ways by which we can deal with a condescending pose of philanthropy on the part of medical caregivers. Why not hop on the current bandwagon of patient autonomy and contractual relations as a way of bringing patients back into the game of medical decision making? May is not entirely opposed to such moves. He sees them as useful correctives in certain times and places. But he is persuaded that covenant — not contract or autonomy — is the internal meaning of creation, the goal toward which we ought to struggle in the moral bonds that claim us. And, in particular, he suggests that contractualism may be less than adequate as a way of regularizing the bond between patients and physicians. For one thing, there is an asymmetry between patient and physician. They are not two equally skillful buyers or sellers meeting in the marketplace; knowledge and power are almost entirely on the side of the professional. Internal checks, cut into the characters of physicians, will be needed (1986a: 6). Moreover, there is a second reason why the bond of patient and physician ought not be reduced to transaction alone: it must be oriented to the patient's deeper needs. It may often call not just for a transaction but for a transformation of the patient's life. If this talk treads dangerously close to a kind of physician paternalism that is objectionable, May thinks it a risk we must take — but a risk whose greatest dangers can be avoided if physicians think of themselves as teachers who bring about needed transformations in patients through teaching rather than deception (1986a: 7-8). There is a third reason, most important of all, why the bond of patient and physician should not become purely contractual. Seeing this reason, we see the complexities of May's position. He has attacked the posture of the physician as self-sufficient, philanthropic caregiver, but he does not wish to ignore the element of the *gratuitous* that must be present. Contractualism reduces the patient-physician bond to obligations that can be codified; it thereby encourages minimalism.[5] But the needs of patients

5. It may also — and this is no better — lead to defensive medicine and maximalism in medical care (1975: 35).

cannot be exhaustively listed in advance, nor are good physicians those who do no more than is contractually required. May writes,

> The professions must be ready to cope with the contingent, the un-expected. Calls upon services may be required that exceed those anticipated in a contract or for which compensation may be available in a given case. These services, moreover, are more likely to be effective in achieving the desired therapeutic result if they are delivered in the context of a fiduciary relationship that the patient or client can really trust. (1975: 34)

The complexity of this view should be evident. Consider what it means to think of medicine as a covenanted profession. On the one hand, physicians should not imagine themselves self-sufficient philanthropists who love without ties; they should know that they are responding to debts when they offer care. On the other hand, they should not become mere contractualists who do only what is required; they should give freely and generously of their skill, time, energy, and wealth in professing medically. They should be philanthropic without assuming the posture of the philanthropist or adopting the sort of ethic (in particular, a cost-benefit ethic) that is "chiefly an ethic for benefactors" (1980a: 362).

How can we have it both ways? Only, May suggests, by remembering that the original location of covenant language is in relation to the transcendent. Even when physicians give philanthropically far more than they have received from their patients and community, they always remain indebted, for they are needy creatures who have been graced by God. "Thus action which at a human level appears gratuitous, in that it is not provoked by a specific gratuity from another human being, is at its deepest level but gift answering to gift" (1975: 36).

Hard Cases

I have noted that May's strength lies not in the exploration of hard cases but in the discussion of background beliefs that shape the vision we bring to such cases. We ought not, however, underestimate the importance of deciding about hard cases or the help that moral codes can render. There might well be circumstances in which I would rather have as my physician someone of relatively impoverished literary or metaphysical insight who had nonetheless been brought up to believe that "a gentleman does not lie," than someone who had as an undergraduate gone almost without sleep for a week while working through various interpretations of Dostoevsky's "Grand Inquisitor." Therefore, having sketched May's vision of ethics and having discussed two themes (the sacral power of death and the meaning of covenant) absolutely central in his work, we will conclude by following his argument on two hard cases.

One of his widely acclaimed articles, "Attitudes Toward the Newly Dead," is in my judgment a very successful application of his approach to a difficult problem in biomedical ethics. The problem is a straightforward one, and it continues to be pressing today. As organ transplantation becomes increasingly possible and successful, the need for organs becomes greater. Available organs may save lives, and modern medicine's salvific urge is not to be gainsaid. Yet the supply of organs — at least when we rely on voluntary donation — is not everything that some might wish. Hence there are arguments about alternative ways of obtaining organs for transplant.

May is fairly quick to rule out one possible approach — the sale of organs by the family of the deceased person or even by the predeceased person himself or herself. Having discussed above May's view of the limits of contractualism, we are hardly surprised that he should believe human organs are not simply "commodities" to be bartered in the market. And more generally, in fact, he tends to agree with those who argue that in matters so fundamental "encouraging a pattern of *giving* will have positive moral consequences for the society at large" (1973: 4). But even with this method ruled out, several options remain. The central argument pits advocates of a "program of organized giving of organs . . . dependent upon the consent of the donor or his family" against proponents of a "system of routine salvaging of organs from which exemption may be granted" only for those who specifically seek it (1973: 4). In "Attitudes Toward the Newly Dead" May argues a fairly modest thesis: "that a system of organized giving must be granted a serious test before entertaining the alternative of routine salvaging" (1973: 4).

Why make such an argument at all, especially if these organs are desperately needed for transplant? After all, we are talking about donors who are corpses, not still living beings. Why the tentativeness and caution? We should know by now that May is not likely to imagine dealing with a dead body an uneventful occurrence. The body, though dead, was the locus of a person's presence, a person bound through that body to others. And death is a power that we naturally fear and avoid. Anyone who felt no horror, who did not shrink back from the dead, would be less than human. May calls to mind a story of the Brothers Grimm — of a young boy incapable of horror, who does not shrink from the dead and even tries to play with a corpse. His father sends him away "to learn how to shudder" (1973: 5). True, we may be deluged with seemingly humanitarian arguments about the need for organs, about the lives that can be saved thereby. But we must remember that the arch-humanist is the Grand Inquisitor, who becomes a savior figure out of his despair at human suffering. "There is a tinge of the inhuman in the humanitarianism of those who believe that the perception of social need easily overrides all other considerations and reduces the acts of implementation to the everyday, routine, and casual" (1973: 5). May notes perceptively the way in which the argument for routine salvaging must, in fact, indirectly acknowledge the horror one ought to feel at it. Asking for consent, we are told by advocates of routine salvaging, is "ghoulish," since it forces us to further trouble those who have just suffered great loss. But why is it ghoulish, May wonders, unless deeper and more fundamental concerns than costs and benefits are involved? (1973: 5).

To explain the difficulty with proposals for routine salvaging, May turns to myth and ritual. Death has often been understood as Hider and Devourer (associations still present in our language, as when we talk of a "consuming disease"). And the hospital, where people in our society go to die, has begun to acquire the image of a place where people are swallowed up. A system of routine salvaging, May argues, would only reinforce these mythic associations — the hospital, where disease is hidden away, would also become quite literally the devourer, the "arch-symbol of a world that devours. . . . One's very vitals must be inventoried, extracted and distributed by the state on behalf of the social order" (1973: 6). This cannot, May argues, be good for the healing professions.

Not only professionals but families are involved. A system of routine salvaging would permit a family to seek exemption from such salvaging and, in that sense, it would not reduce the dead person to a mere part of the social whole. But May reflects on the meaning of such a requirement for the family. The ritual of the funeral service functions in several ways. It reinforces the continuity between the person now dead and his or her family; yet it also acknowledges publicly that this continuity has been broken (1973: 7). In Sophocles' tragedy *Antigone*, Creon's crime is not simply that he claims the body of Polyneices as his own, but that he compels Antigone to claim as her own possession the body of the brother whom death has forced her to surrender (1973: 8).

This is only a partial summary of the reasons May offers in defense of his claim that a system of organized giving is preferable to one of routine salvaging and that such a system deserves a fair test. He goes on to suggest that there are excellent reasons within Christian theology to encourage organ donation, but I will not follow the argument further here. More than a decade later May returned to the topic in "Religious Justifications for Donating Body Parts" (1985b). His argument remained essentially the same, but I think we see more clearly in the second essay what is at stake for May. Twelve years after the original argument had been made, one might claim that the fair test May thought necessary had been made and a system of organized giving found inadequate. That May does not reach such a conclusion suggests to me that his initial argument was more far-reaching than his own language implied. He was not really asking simply for a trial of one system before turning to another. He was arguing that a society would be better — more humane in its sensitivity to the significance of the human body, in its respect for the covenants that bind human beings in families, in its resolute determination to avoid the temptation to make medicine salvific, and in its recognition of the extraterritoriality of the human person in relation to the social order — if it eschewed a system of routine salvaging even when a simple cost-benefit calculus seemed to recommend it. Better than such "mandated universal routine" would be continued effort to encourage social institutions and religious communities to use their powerful symbolic force to encourage the giving of organs for transplant (1985b: 38). Here is an instance in which May has turned his entire armamentarium on a hard case, explored it insightfully, illuminated it richly, and argued powerfully for a particular resolution.

I conclude with a second example, though one in which May is, I think, less successful. In "Dealing with Catastrophe" (1989) May examines the well-known Texas burn case of Donald (Dax) Cowart. He argues that attempts to analyze it and make ethical judgments about appropriate treatment in terms of "life versus quality of life" are shallow.

The truth is, he suggests, that Donald Cowart's life was not just modified and changed by his accident; it was annihilated. Donald Cowart has died (1989: 133). In part this judgment rests on May's general sense that we *are* our bodies. And in a case such as this one, the body has been so altered and shattered that it can no longer be a mode of self-revelation for the same self. The body is also our means of mastering and savoring the world. But Dax has suffered "a permanent alteration in ability to master, control, and enjoy the world" (1989: 138). Because he "looks" so different, he has *become* different. "The patient's 'look' is not an abstract object of aesthetic judgment. It is always *someone's* look and therefore cuts to the core of *self*-presentation. An alien has now taken over that presentation" (1989: 139-40).

It is important — but perhaps worrisome — that May presses the argument considerably beyond cases involving severe disfigurement of the body, and one wonders whether in so doing May has not moved too far beyond the points often made in his writing about the significance of the body. He argues in this essay that any serious blow to the ties or connections of our life may be equally decisive metaphysically. "The highway accident, the devastating fire, the mental breakdown of a family member, the irreversible, progressive, and immobilizing disease transform the substance of one's existence; they do not merely qualify life at its edges" (1989: 141).

In any case, unless and until we see this ultimate connection of the body to the self, we are bound, May thinks, to make a "series of false assumptions" (1989: 141). Putting the issue in terms of life versus quality of life, we move quickly to debates about who should decide (autonomy versus paternalism). But if this is no longer the same life, the same person — if we are dealing with something other than changed quality of a subsisting individual — these categories may not be helpful. Instead, we should think in terms of death and rebirth, asking what responsibilities we have toward Dax Cowart now that Donald Cowart is dead. As May remarks, "If there is any life after such events, it will depend upon radical reconstruction from the ground up. . ." (1989: 142).

It is puzzling that in his attempt to shift the categories away from stale arguments pitting autonomy against paternalism, May turns to what is essentially the language of self-creation. Of patients in such circumstances he writes, "They shape their own narrative" (1989: 146). Certainly there is an appropriate place for such language about the decisions through which we determine the person we are and will be. Yet it omits much of what one expects from May — of the self as existing in its relationships and bonds, of the relationship to sacral powers. May rejects the analogy that would depict such a patient as a newborn, in need of parental and paternal care (1989: 148-49).[6] Yet his apparent metaphysical claim makes the analogy plausible. Why speak of self-creation here apart from the context of all-enveloping parental care and decision making? He rejects the idea that we should ask whether it is proper to let such a patient die — since, after all, he *has* died. But does that help? Don't we then simply find ourselves asking whether this new patient, with his or her particular set of circumstances, should be allowed to die? In short, in this instance May's attempt to set a hard case into a larger, richer context does not seem finally to illuminate the decisions that must be made.

"Dealing with Catastrophe" *does* make some perfectly sensible recommendations — for example, that we need to invest more heavily in rehabilitative and chronic care (1989: 145). But we hardly needed the metaphysical jolt May has given us to arrive at that conclusion. May's effort to paint the big picture has also tempted him into some less compelling recommendations — for example, that we have not done what we ought if we only protect a trauma victim's life without enabling him or her to reconstruct it. "The language of life/death/rebirth . . . makes it clear that the responsibility of the community has just begun if it has imposed continuance upon the individual in the midst of what the individual can only experience as a living death" (1989: 145).

At one level this statement is obviously true. But at another level it ignores the distinction between negative and positive duties — our duty not to harm and our duty to bring aid in a variety of ways. Even if in some circumstances we cannot bring all the aid we might wish or all the aid that is needed, this does not release us from the obligation not to do harm — not, at least, unless we give in to the temptation of the Grand Inquisitor and try simply to eliminate as much suffering as we can.

Whatever we make of such judgments about hard cases, however, there is no denying that anyone proposing to think about bioethics will be richly rewarded by study of the writing of William F. May. The range and catholicity of his intellect, and the grace of his writing, make him

6. This formulation is eliminated in *The Patient's Ordeal* (1991).

unlike anyone else currently writing on these topics. If we would not go first to his work for an unpacking of twelve different approaches to a single hard case, we would and should go to his work — perhaps first to his work — to learn how to think about what makes any case hard. And always, we will learn as well something of what it means to think theologically, to let our ethical vision be corrected and transformed by the insights of Christian theology. To him there is nothing human — story, myth, symbol, ritual — that is alien. But to him there is also nothing human that is not in need of correction and transformation when related to the transcendence of God.

References

Barth, Karl. 1958. *Church Dogmatics,* III/1. Edinburgh: T. and T. Clark.

Capron, Alexander Morgan. 1986. "In Praise of William May's 'Attitudes.'" *Hastings Center Report* 16, no. 5: 8-9.

Feinberg, Joel. 1985. "The Mistreatment of Dead Bodies." *Hastings Center Report* 15, no. 1: 31-37.

May, William F. 1969. "The Sacral Power of Death in Contemporary Experience." In *Perspectives on Death,* ed. Liston D. Mills, 168-96. Nashville: Abingdon.

————. 1972. "The Sacral Power of Death in Contemporary Experience." *Social Research* 39: 463-88.

————. 1973. "Attitudes Toward the Newly Dead." *Hastings Center Studies* 1: 3-13.

————. 1974. "The Metaphysical Plight of the Family." *Hastings Center Studies* 2: 19-30.

————. 1975. "Code, Covenant, Contract, or Philanthropy." *Hastings Center Report* 5: 29-38.

————. 1976. "Institutions as Symbols of Death." *Journal of the American Academy of Religion* 44: 211-23.

————. 1980a. "Doing Ethics: The Bearing of Ethical Theories on Fieldwork." *Social Problems* 27: 358-70.

————. 1980b. "Professional Ethics: Setting, Terrain and Teacher." In *Ethics Teaching in Higher Education,* ed. Daniel Callahan and Sissela Bok, 205-41. New York: Plenum.

————. 1981. "Response to Farley." *Journal of Supervision and Training in Ministry* 4: 121-34.

————. 1982a. "A Public Justification for the Liberal Arts." *Liberal Education* 68: 285-96.

————. 1982b. "Who Cares for the Elderly?" *Hastings Center Report* 12: 31-37.

————. 1983a. "Parenting, Bonding and Valuing the Retarded Child." In *Natural Abilities and Perceived Worth: Rights, Values, and Retarded Persons,* ed. Loretta Kopelman and John Moskop, 141-60. Dordrecht, Netherlands: D. Reidel.

————. 1983b. *The Physician's Covenant: Images of the Healer in Medical Ethics.* Philadelphia: Westminster.

————. 1984a. "The Virtues in a Professional Setting." In *Annual of the Society of Christian Ethics,* ed. Larry Rasmussen, 71-91. Vancouver: Vancouver School of Theology.

————. 1984b. "Why Theology and Religious Studies Need Each Other." *Journal of the American Academy of Religion* 52: 748-57.

————. 1985a. "The Virtues and Vices of the Elderly." *Socio-Economic Planning Sciences* 19: 255-62.

————. 1985b. "Religious Justifications for Donating Body Parts." *Hastings Center Report* 15: 38-42.

————. 1986a. *Professional Responsibility: Law, Medicine, and Clergy.* Dallas: Southern Methodist University.

————. 1986b. "Professional Ethics, the University, and the Journalist." *Journal of Mass Media Ethics* 1: 20-31.

————. 1988. "Four Mischievous Theories of Sex: Casual, Demonic, Divine, and Nuisance." In *Passionate Attachments: Thinking About Love,* ed. Willard Gaylin and Ethel Person, 27-39. New York: Free Press.

————. 1989. "Dealing with Catastrophe." In *Dax's Case: Essays in Medical Ethics and Human Meaning,* ed. Lonnie D. Kliever, 131-50. Dallas: Southern Methodist University Press.

————. 1991. *The Patient's Ordeal.* Bloomington and Indianapolis: Indiana University Press.

Ramsey, Paul. 1970. *The Patient as Person.* New Haven and London: Yale University Press.

Veatch, Robert M. 1986. "Challenging the Power of Codes." *Hastings Center Report* 16, no. 5: 14-15.

ON JAMES F. CHILDRESS

Answering That of God in Every Person

COURTNEY S. CAMPBELL

MANY THEOLOGIANS in the field of medical ethics believe that their primary vocational responsibility is to be faithful to a theological tradition and responsive to particular religious communities. This fidelity requires that the religious dimensions and theological perspectives of ethical issues be articulated explicitly and forcefully. Not to do so is to risk forfeiting theological integrity and even professional credibility.[1]

The medical ethics of James F. Childress makes it clear that the boundaries of the community of ethical responsibility should not be drawn too narrowly. The prominent theological theme in Quaker thought (Childress's tradition) of "answering that of God in every person" carries a universalistic impulse, requiring the ethicist to take account of and be accountable to nontheologically informed positions. The responsibility to answer to a community constituted by "every person" may entail a less explicit, background role for theological convictions in moral discourse. As in Childress's case, there may be *theological* reasons for not doing medical ethics theologically.

---

1. I have briefly summarized the central objections forcefully articulated by James M. Gustafson (1978: 386-92) to religious ethicists who fail to make explicit the religious dimensions of their positions. According to Gustafson, the choice for such persons is clear: "They will either have to become moral philosophers with a special interest in 'religious' texts and arguments, or become theologians," developing their positions out of and in response to "historically identifiable religious communities."

For Childress, the metaphor of "answering" nevertheless clarifies the role of justification in ethics, the relation of God to the world, and the nature of moral agency. In this essay, I will highlight the role of such theological considerations and indicate their relation to other influential sources of Childress's ethics, thereby illuminating their implications for his ethical method. We will then consider how this method works in four topics in which Childress has been an especially prominent figure: respect for autonomy and paternalism, the forgoing of medical nutrition and hydration for terminally ill patients, the rationing of scarce lifesaving medical resources, and public policies for organ procurement.

I. Answering: Moral Responsibility and Justification

It should be acknowledged at the outset that Childress's ethics is marked more by a syncretistic and pluralistic approach than by a dominant reliance on one tradition of thought. His ideas of responsibility and justification in the moral life have been explicitly shaped by patterns of legal reasoning. Similarly, his interpretation of moral norms and their status has been heavily influenced by philosophical traditions of ethics, particularly that articulated by analytic philosophers such as W. D. Ross. In each of these instances, however, theological perspectives also have played an indirect role as background, buttressing assumptions.

A major theme in recent theological and philosophical ethics is responsibility.[2] The key questions for such an ethic are responsibility *to whom* and *for what*. In his work in both medical and social ethics, Childress considers the concept of "moral justification" to be integral to any account of responsibility in the moral life. Justification is a form of "answering" that involves "the appeal to moral principles, rules, and values to defeat charges of moral liability" (1983a: 276, 278; 1982b). Indeed, part of what it means to be a moral agent is to assume responsibility to others for justifying one's actions. The claims of conscience, other persons, and God are answered by giving reasons to validate conduct.

2. The classic exposition of an "ethics of responsibility" was articulated by Max Weber in his essay "Politics as a Vocation" (1958: 77-128). More recently, such prominent figures as H. Richard Niebuhr (1963) and Hans Jonas (1984) have developed their ethical positions around the concept of responsibility.

While the metaphors of "appeal," "charges," and "liability" reveal the influence of legal reasoning, Childress's interpretation of moral justification is likewise shaped by and critiques theological perspectives. In particular, the metaphor of "answering," articulated in the ethics of seventeenth-century Quaker thinker George Fox, is a supporting theological source of Childress's account. Fox's idea of "answering that of God in every person" emphasizes responsiveness to the directions of the Spirit. This view may seem initially at odds with a stress on justification of one's action *to others*. However, Childress contends that the Quaker understanding is much more complex than a simple recommendation of theological intuitionism: The content of "that of God" includes norms such as the unity of mankind, natural affections, the primitive order, humanity, and ordering to the glory of God (1974). For Fox, these provide standards to which every person must answer; "answering" is thus compatible with and analogous to moral reasoning.

Legal models of responsibility as well as Fox's theology of answering are incorporated by Childress to suggest several elements of an account of moral justification. First, answering, as a response that evokes a response from the other, conveys continuity and dialogue in moral discourse. Second, the evoked response will confirm or invalidate one's answer depending on the appropriateness of the reasons advanced (1974: 13, 30). Finally, "answering . . . every person" implies that the process of moral justification is universal, encompassing both its participants and its audience. In this respect, moral justification reflects a fundamental claim about our common humanity and expresses part of what it means to be *social* beings (1971: 167).

This interpretation of moral justification is developed *against* other theological perspectives, in particular the traditional Protestant suspicion of the language of "moral justification." Protestants claim that God and God alone justifies human beings, that is, accepts them as righteous, even though they are not righteous. Hence justification as an activity that *we* engage in may be viewed as encroaching on the sovereignty and freedom of God. Moreover, moral justification could be construed as a form of "works-righteousness" in which the decisive criterion of the righteousness of the agent is the conformity of his or her conduct to prescribed rules and requirements. The freedom of the believer to act with creativity and imagination seems infringed when we impose standards and consequences for moral judgment (1971: 165, 166; 1983a: 278). A model of ethics that gives primacy to moral justification, then, may risk "legalism," in which adherence to rules and laws is the center of the moral life.

Childress argues, however, that analogies with law do not necessarily lead to legalism. Nor is he convinced that theological suspicion of moral justification is entirely warranted. There may be continuity between moral and religious justification, for example, in assessing the relationship between right conduct and right character. In addition, moral justification "does not eliminate the need for God's grace or limit God's freedom" (1983a: 278; 1986d: 332-33).

Moral Standards and Principles

If moral justification means that we answer to others for our actions relative to certain norms or standards, what, it must be asked, might these standards be? Childress's ethical method identifies five major principles comprising an "embedded common morality" (1989b: 88), which may be defended and accepted on theological or nontheological grounds.

The principle of *nonmaleficence* prohibits the infliction of harm, injury, or death upon others. This principle is closely associated with the maxim *primum non nocere* (above all, or at least, do no harm) in the Hippocratic medical tradition, and is a necessary, even if minimal, component of *agape* or love of neighbor. However, Childress also contends that nonmaleficence is a "bedrock of social morality" and "human interaction" (1986f: 425); its status therefore does not depend on theological premises.

Nonmaleficence must be supplemented, however, since we are also positively engaged in seeking to promote the welfare of others. The principle of *beneficence* includes actions that prevent and remove harm as well as doing good toward them. In the Hippocratic tradition, the principle of "patient benefit" reflects beneficence, and indeed is the fundamental rationale for medical care.

Beneficence also overlaps with *agape* but does not exhaust its meaning. For example, many philosophical positions maintain that a duty to assist is morally mandatory only when such actions carry minimal risk or inconvenience to the agent, whereas *agape* is usually understood to involve some sacrifice of the agent's interests. For Childress, *agape* may require more but certainly never less than beneficence (1982c: 34-37).

Since it is not always possible to avoid inflicting harm while doing good, we frequently must balance the benefits and harms of an action. The principle of *utility,* Childress holds, requires us to seek the action that will produce the greatest benefit over harm. While the most philosophically refined defenses of this principle are found in utilitarian moral theories, Childress believes that its moral meaning can be expressed theologically in the principle of proportionality, or proportionate good (1986j: 512).

The principles of nonmaleficence, beneficence, and utility are united by a moral concern for orienting action in ways that achieve the optimal consequences, ends, or results. By contrast, two other fundamental principles, *justice* and *respect for persons,* place moral constraints on the means used to achieve desired results. These principles have independent standing and in certain circumstances can conflict with *agape*. On this latter point, Childress disagrees with the late Protestant ethicist Paul Ramsey, who maintained that justice (as well as all other moral norms) is a second-order principle that derives from love (Smith 1987).

While the principle of utility has to do with the aggregate balance of benefits and burdens, justice concerns how these are distributed among various social groups and individuals. Justice requires fairness in allocating benefits and burdens. If a proposed policy appears to have enormous aggregate benefits, but would impose a disproportionate share of burdens on identified groups or persons, it violates justice.

The fundamental meaning Childress ascribes to the principle of respect for persons is that "it is [prima facie] wrong to subject the actions (including choices) of others to controlling influence" (1990b: 13). His interpretation is strongly influenced by the German philosopher Immanuel Kant's second formulation of his categorical imperative: "Act so that you treat humanity, whether in your own person or in that of another, always as an end and never as a means only" (Kant 1969: 54; Childress 1987a: 28), and likewise draws on theological and philosophical traditions of reflection on respect for conscience (1979a: 315-35; Beauchamp and Childress 1989: 385-94). Indeed, Childress has acknowledged that the "roots" of his interest in questions of conscience and disassociation from evil, subissues of what it means to respect persons as ends, may be found in the Quaker tradition (1990a: 32).

While respect for persons is independent of *agape,* it does not always "win" in case of conflict, nor is it "the single, exclusive, or overriding principle of biomedical ethics" (Childress 1984a: 31). Childress argues that while love without respect is demeaning, absolute priority of respect for persons over beneficence risks apathy and neglect. Caregivers are obliged to seek a proper balance between care and concern and respect to avoid the alternative "temptations" of indignity and indifference (1982c: ix; 1986i: 451).

This moral requirement to respect the wishes, choices, and actions of other persons may nonetheless pose real and difficult conflicts with *agape* and the obligations of health care professionals to benefit their patients. Childress illustrates this conflict by reconceiving the parable of the good Samaritan, the biblical narrative often considered the paradigm case of neighbor-love (Luke 10:30-37). If, when the Samaritan came upon the wounded traveler, the injured person had refused assistance and indicated a desire to die, what should the Samaritan have done? By analogy, how should medical professionals respond when patients choose to forgo medical treatment? Even though love might require the kinds of actions related in the parable, respect might entail accepting the person's request (Childress 1985: 225-26).[3]

Metaphors and Moral Imagination

While the ethic of principles advocated by Childress (and others) has been the target of substantial criticism in bioethics recently, it is important to note that Childress has consistently devoted attention to the role of metaphors and analogical reasoning as a complement to his discussion of these five normative principles. This emphasis on metaphors balances the responsibility of moral agents to answer for their actions with a stress on persons' capacity for imagination and creativity that helps us "see" or perceive moral dilemmas in the first instance (1982a: 69; Childress and Siegler 1984). As displayed above, it is within this context that Childress incorporates the significance of stories and nar-

3. I have presented a very compressed version of some of the major themes in Beauchamp and Childress (1989: 25-306), although it is important to note a couple of differences. I have distinguished beneficence and utility as separate principles, whereas in *Principles of Biomedical Ethics*, utility is considered one aspect of the principle of beneficence. I have also used the language of respect for persons rather than respect for autonomy. In both instances, these distinctions seem more representative of Childress's own moral framework, as contrasted with that articulated in a jointly authored text. Where possible, I have directed readers to alternative sources to support this interpretation.

ratives in traditions, both religious and professional, of moral discourse. While normative principles provide the grounds or justification of an obligation, metaphors and stories, like the good Samaritan parable, can enable the *recognition* of an obligation (1983a: 279).

While Childress has not developed this dimension of his ethics fully, one example should suffice to show the interrelationship between moral principles and moral imagination. Childress has illustrated how pervasive an understanding of "medicine as warfare" is in contemporary health care. This way of seeing medicine has considerable moral import, for "the military metaphor tends to assign priority to health care . . . over other goods and, within health care, to critical interventions over prevention and chronic care, killer over disabling diseases, technological interventions over care, and heroic treatment of dying patients" (1984a: 30, 31). Some of these priorities may be supported by moral principles, such as nonmaleficence or beneficence, while others are open to sharp criticism from principles of utility, justice, or respect for persons.

Moral Conflict and Prudence

This raises the question of how, in a case of conflict between principles, a person can decide which principle "wins." On Childress's account, the answer depends on how such principles are understood to function in moral justification. Childress rejects three alternatives that have been influential in Christian theological ethics: (1) one principle (for example, love) is superordinate and absolute; (2) several principles are arranged in a prioritized order; (3) moral principles illuminate but do not prescribe; they are maxims without normative force. Drawing heavily on W. D. Ross's account, Childress instead advocates a pluralist method: Each principle is *prima facie* or presumptively obligatory, but none possesses a pre-assigned priority. In a concrete case of moral conflict, moreover, any principle can be overridden by competing principles (1986g: 425-27; Beauchamp and Childress 1989: 44-55).

A determination of which principle "wins" in a moral dilemma involves also what Childress refers to as the "moral logic of prima facie duties." This logic is substantially indebted to the form of moral reasoning displayed in arguments about the morality of resorting to lethal violence, particularly as articulated in the just war tradition that has been prominent in Christian social ethics. Childress contends: "We formulate and use criteria that are analogous to those that determine whether a war is just or justified *whenever* we face conflicting obligations or duties, whenever it is impossible to fulfill all the claims upon us, to respect all the rights involved, or to avoid doing evil to everyone" (1982b: 66-67; my emphasis). A decision to override the principle of respect for persons (what will be described below as the conflict of paternalism), for example, must satisfy conditions of proportionality, effectiveness, last resort, and least infringement (1990b: 15) — all of which are formal criteria in the just war tradition.

This reliance on a logic of moral reasoning is once again balanced by, and perhaps in tension with, the interpretations and experience of moral agents. "The practical application of principles and rules is not mechanical since it presupposes discernment and prudence" (1986g: 427; 1989c: 41). It is therefore simply mistaken to assume that ethical decisions can be reduced to the precision of a formula or that an ethic of principles is necessarily abstract and alien to the everyday, lived-in world. Childress's approach clearly implies methodological sensitivity to human experience and the need for a dialectical and corrective relationship between ethical theory and ordinary moral experience and judgments. Nevertheless, Childress has yet to develop fully an account of practical reasoning that shows how to distinguish adequately between discernment and prudence and mere arbitrary intuitions or personal preferences.

This suggests a significant limitation to the pluralist method. Childress's rationale for adopting this method, along with the procedural moral logic that reduces but does not eliminate its intuitional elements, requires that we attend to some of its theological and anthropological underpinnings.

II. That of God: Theology and Ethics

Childress concurs with neoorthodox theologian H. Richard Niebuhr that a determination of "what is going on" in a situation of moral conflict can be shaped by theological convictions about the doctrine of God (1981: 102-4). Moral perception of a situation may then be expressed theologically in the question, "What is God doing?" (H. R. Niebuhr 1942: 630; 1963: 60-65, 126).

For Childress, the metaphor of answering structures our understanding of what God is doing in the world and how we are to respond.

In our capacity to "answer" to claims upon us, we are responsive to "that of God in every person." What is God doing to which we as moral selves are accountable? In his social ethics, Childress has followed Paul Ramsey (and thus H. Richard Niebuhr) in contending that an adequate Christian ethics requires the "whole idea" of God. That is, divine purposive activity can and theologically must be understood in terms of creating, ordering (including both sustaining and restraining), and redeeming. While these purposes are finally inseparable, they and human responses to them can be differentiated (1971: 101, 102). Theological ethics is challenged not only to affirm all three aspects of divine purpose, but to balance them.

This understanding of the doctrine of God, Childress claims, supports a pluralist model for ethical reflection. "[A] pluralist approach is most consistent with an adequate, balanced understanding of God's creative, ruling, and redeeming will" (1971: 103). Two significant implications follow from this claim. First, the plurality of the divine nature correlates with an ethical method that draws on a multiplicity of moral principles. Second, the balance required in reflecting the three dimensions of divine purpose theologically buttresses Childress's position on the status and weight of moral principles: In a theologically qualified pluralism, "no single principle or value receives exclusive attention" (1971: 103, 104).

This relation of theological affirmation and ethical method, it must be stressed, is one of correlation rather than derivation. Theological convictions do not, in Childress's view, constitute obligations, that is, they do not furnish the premises from which moral conclusions are then derived, nor is faith a necessary condition of morality. Rather, theology provides ethics with an interpretative framework or perspective that illuminates relevant moral obligations (1981: 102-4; 1983a: 279, 285-86), obligations that already may be accepted by nonbelievers on nontheological grounds. For example, an understanding of God's impartial loving care for human beings can illuminate the moral priority of equality in the allocation of resources.

There are also important limits to this theological-ethical correlativity. The ultimate inseparability of the triune divine nature has no analogical counterpart at the level of Childress's practical ethics. Unlike Ramsey, for example, Childress does not hold that all moral principles can be derived from one supreme norm, such as love. Because the normative principles of Childress's ethics are independent rather than derivative, they come into conflict. Childress's method therefore at least theoretically accommodates genuine moral dilemmas and even moral tragedy, irresolvable conflicts of moral obligations.

III. In Every Person: Human Nature and Ethics

God's activity, expressed theologically as creating, ordering, and redeeming, may also, according to Childress, be expressed in correlative anthropological terms: Human beings can be understood as created, fallen, and redeemed. A coherent ethics must account for these dimensions of human nature and attempt to hold them in balance and tension. Two themes with deep roots in theological ethics, the *imago dei* (image of God) and sin, have important implications in Childress's normative ethics.

That human beings are part of nature, Childress contends, is reflected in their earthly creatureliness and in their status as created beings. But human beings are also a unique part of nature, as illumined in scripture, created in the image of God (1981: 103, 104). For Childress (following Reinhold Niebuhr), *imago Dei*, which expresses "that of God in every person" means in part that human beings possess the capacity for self-transcendence, that we can consider more than a narrow pursuit of our own self-interest (1986c: 292-93). This capacity is a necessary condition for moral discourse. If persons as moral agents are to answer to each other, they must recognize and respect others' interests and ends.

The *imago Dei* also means that human beings have "dominion over nature," understood as "stewardship, trusteeship, or administration" (1989a: 230, 239). Yet however elevated human beings may be relative to the rest of creation, we still remain only an image of the divine nature. Our created status implies ontological limits to our powers and capacities, which are experienced frequently in our limited capabilities to predict, control, and assess our actions (in contrast to divine omniscience, omnipotence, and infallibility). Finitude and moral fallibility are as much a part of the human condition as self-transcendence (1981: 118; 1982b: 57-61).

Human sinfulness, displayed as a notorious tendency for self-interestedness, for seeking our own good at the expense of others, imposes additional limits of moral significance. Our problem, according to Childress, is not simply that finitude inhibits reflection, but also that our predictions, capacity for control, and moral assessments persistently favor personal interests and needs. Self-interestedness likewise infects our judgments, diminishing the efficacy of moral reasoning, persuasion, and answering.

These background beliefs about human nature[4] inform Childress's ethics in important ways. The theme of *imago Dei*, for example, theologically grounds several important moral principles, including respect for persons. As beings created in the image of God, persons deserve and demand respect from others. They are not to be treated merely as means, and the reasons they give for actions should be taken seriously.

Childress connects the respect for persons principle with this theological claim to distinguish it from the principle of autonomy. Respect for persons cannot be "reduced to the modern liberal conception of autonomy, because its religious context includes embodiment, not merely personal choices, and also limits set by God" (1989a: 230; 1986a: 51). The language of autonomy is too easily identified with an ideology of unfettered individualism and moral minimalism. Thus, while the political ideology of Anglo-American liberalism may identify autonomy with self-determination limited only by equal self-determination for others, from a theological perspective autonomy must be qualified by considerations of dependence, sociality, and finitude.

The theme of *imago Dei*, furthermore, presents a fundamental moral claim that all persons be treated as equals. In addition, "beliefs about God's creation and redemption of human life (e.g., God created human beings in his image) are claims about humanity that can support a right to life" (1986e: 131; 1989a: 231).

Though we are created in the image of God, Childress does not believe we have the capacity to imitate God in our moral decision making. Human finitude and fallibility warrant particular suspicion of consequentialist moral theories, which are typically too idealistic about human nature. Even if God is a utilitarian, as the Anglican theologian Joseph Butler once speculated (1983: 74-75), Childress is quite clear that human beings have few grounds for adopting such a moral stance.

---

4. Childress's moral anthropology has been profoundly influenced by the thought of Reinhold Niebuhr (1964), mitigating some of the optimism and idealism about human nature associated with the Quaker tradition. Niebuhr's political "realism" and emphasis on human sinfulness were instrumental in converting Childress from a pacifist to a defender of just war theory.

The complexity of the moral life is due not only to human limitations in determining the right or the good, but also to inabilities in performing it. The pervasiveness of sin and moral weakness presents an important test of adequacy of any ethical method. Childress accounts for this "fact" of human nature in at least two ways. First, the dimension of finitude, fallibility, and sin support a rule-governed conception of the moral life. Moral principles and rules are necessary in part to compensate for human tendencies to rationalize and engage in self-interested action. They establish obligations, without which such tendencies might lead to antinomianism ("no law") and moral anarchy. When defended as moral absolutes, principles and rules risk moral tyranny and legalism, Childress concedes, but given the darker side of the human condition, it is more realistic to fear *most* the situation of moral anarchy (1986k: 586-88).

These convictions about human nature likewise indicate a prominent role for procedures in moral decision making. Moral reasoning, accountability, and institutional standards provide a basis for moral interaction in a pluralistic society where disagreement exists over the values that ought to direct decisions and actions (1984b: 59; 1989c: 42-43).

This claim takes on added significance against the backdrop of current debates in theological and philosophical ethics, in which the importance of community is frequently affirmed over against the individualism of a liberal societal ethos. According to such views, community is based on trust and shared substantive values, while liberal individualism supports only the most minimal moral culture whose members, if they interact at all, relate only as "strangers."

While Childress does not deny the moral significance of community, he believes the dichotomy of community versus individual is misleading. If proponents of the dichotomy were consistent, they would ultimately be forced to claim that moral discourse between members of different communities and traditions is an illusion. Childress is not willing to concede that moral discourse in a pluralistic society is meaningless because a shared commitment to certain procedural values exists. Pluralism does not preclude meaningful moral relations between "friendly strangers," whose bond may be a commitment, expressed in support for fair procedures, to treat others as equals (1980: 38).

This contextual argument for procedures is supplemented by one that roots procedures in human nature. Procedures enable decision makers to respond more adequately to human limitations. Because of our limited predictive capabilities, there are no guarantees that the results of our actions will be fair and just (1981: 118). We can, however, establish and implement fair procedures. Thus, for example, in a situation where scarce resources must be rationed and we can neither predict the outcome of rationing nor agree on how to achieve it, we can at least affirm a fundamental equality among prospective recipients by establishing a procedural method of randomness.

Furthermore, while they do not eradicate sin, procedures can minimize its impact on the moral life (1981: 103). Procedures can counter the bias that afflicts moral decision making and its potential for imposing a self-interested vision of the human good on others who do not share such a vision. Given the universality of sin in human experience, Childress contends, it is necessary to "support procedures to prevent one sinful person from overriding the wishes, choices, and actions of another sinful person" (1986i: 450). For Childress, this kind of moral imperialism, and the need to limit it, is exemplified most acutely in conflicts between health care professionals and patients.

IV. Paternalism

The principle of beneficence (as well as the Hippocratic value of patient benefit and the religious norm of *agape*) requires that health care professionals provide care that promotes the welfare of their patients. When patient welfare is emphasized to the exclusion of patient choices, the moral conflict of paternalism arises. As Childress defines it, paternalism is a "refusal to acquiesce in a person's wishes, choices or actions for that person's own benefit" (1982c: vii). Paternalistic actions may include withholding information from a patient; disclosure of information to third parties without patient consent; invasion of a person's body, such as in the provision of life-sustaining treatment, without that person's consent; refusal to carry out a patient request for a medical procedure, such as sterilization or abortion; or provision of unwanted services. Paternalism may also take the form of lying, deception, or even coercion, as in cases of involuntary commitment (1982c: 113).

Paternalism is morally interesting because it is based on an appeal to the welfare, needs, or best interests of the patient. However, to the extent that it overrides patient choices and actions it is prima facie wrong, because acts on the patient's behalf are performed without or against his or her behest. Under certain circumstances, ordinarily benef- icent actions can be demeaning and insulting. In Childress's view, there- fore, it is morally necessary for beneficent action to be constrained by the principle of respect for persons, along the lines of the following image: "[B]eneficence provides the engine — the motivation and direc- tion — of medical care, while the patient's wishes, choices, and actions determine the tracks along which it runs" (Childress and Campbell 1989: 28). On this account, the choices of patients who are competent and able to make autonomous decisions regarding disclosure or non- disclosure of information, refusal of lifesaving medical treatment, or personal life-style should be respected.

The moral logic of paternalism is, according to Childress, suspect for several reasons. A necessary assumption of paternalistic action, that it will enhance patient welfare, is vulnerable to the same critique Childress applies to consequentialist morality generally: "the necessity for prediction and assessment of outcomes . . . tends to undermine paternalism on its own grounds without appeal to other principles of morality" (1982c: 44). The constraints imposed by finitude and falli- bility are sufficient nonmoral reasons to reject paternalism.

Paternalism also raises a question about what constitutes patient need or welfare, or more fundamentally, health. Theological perspectives can support narrow interpretations of these concepts, and consequently, broad views of professional control. Many interpretations of the biblical love commandment, Childress notes, assume an objective or unitary understanding of the neighbor's interests and needs, while the doctrine of sin works to erode the validity of the patient's own interpretation of his or her interests (1982c: 35-39; 1986i: 450, 451). In practice, pro- fessionals and patients will often differ in their views of patient welfare.

The exclusion of the patient's perspective renders paternalism defi- cient on moral grounds. In cases where paternalistic action violates the principle of respect for persons, the patient experiences an assault on his or her dignity:

> [A] professional's refusal to acquiesce in a person's wishes, choices and actions, where no one else is harmed, and merely because the professional disagrees with the values of the patient's life plan and risk budget, is a profound affront to dignity and independence. . . . Paternalism is insulting because it treats the patient as a child, that

is, as one who has not yet freely and competently, and with adequate information, formed a conception of good and evil, of benefits and harms, or is not able to act on that conception in these circumstances. (1982c: 68, 69)

Paternalism is thus sufficiently problematic for Childress because of its inattention both to the decisions of patients and to the values that inform such decisions (1982a: 49-51). Yet, while paternalism may tempt professionals to self-righteousness and the "arrogance of benevolence," critics of paternalism may be tempted by "sloth and indifference." The ethical challenge is to maintain "a tension between the principles of beneficence and respect" (1982c: ix).

This moral tension is expressed in the "principle of limited paternalism," which Childress describes as a "procedural solution to [substantive] conflict about the good" (1986i: 450). Limited paternalism both counters the prevalent paternalistic medical ethos and morally allows paternalism under certain circumstances (1980: 34-35). It specifies actions by which "agents meet the needs of other persons without insulting them" (1982c: 103).

Paternalistic interventions can be justified if five conditions are satisfied: (1) The patient's capacity to express wishes or to act on them must be limited to the extent that his or her competence is questionable; (2) there must be a probability of harm to the patient without paternalistic intervention; (3) the probable benefit to be achieved by intervention must be greater than the probable harm of nonintervention; (4) there must be a reasonable chance that the intervention will achieve the benefit; (5) the intervention should be the least restrictive and humiliating of possible alternatives. If these conditions are satisfied, paternalistic interventions "even against [a] person's express wishes do not signify disrespect or constitute an indignity" (1982c: 102-13; 1990b: 15).

The principle of limited paternalism concisely illustrates the moral logic of prima facie duties at work in Childress's ethical method. Several conditions must be satisfied to justify infringing patient choices, but the moral force of the principle of respect for persons continues to be acknowledged: The "least restrictive" condition, for example, would entail that temporary restriction of action is morally preferable to long-term confinement, and if possible, entail an explanation or justification of the intervention to the person whose action is so limited.

Paternalism and the principles of beneficence and respect for persons set the moral parameters within which Childress addresses the very controversial question of withdrawing one form of medical treatment, artificial nutrition and hydration. His position has been influential not only among professional colleagues, but also for the formulation of public policy, having been cited in precedent-setting court cases on this issue in Massachusetts and New Jersey.

V. Forgoing Medical Nutrition and Hydration

Childress holds that the principles of beneficence and respect for persons each establish a presumption in favor of providing all medical treatment that prolongs life, since prolonging life is typically considered in a patient's interest and also desired by the patient (1986l: 69). However, under certain circumstances, this obligation may be overridden by either principle, for example, when competent patients refuse medical treatment.

But many decisions about terminating medical treatment are made on behalf of incompetent patients who never expressed their treatment preferences, thus underscoring the relevance of the principle of limited paternalism. Childress contends that proxies for the patient should make decisions based on a standard of *best interests,* a patient-centered standard based on beneficence that favors provision of treatment when it has (1) a reasonable chance of success and when (2) successful treatment will realize proportionately greater benefits than burdens for the patient. However, there may be instances when the patient's interests are better served by discontinuing medical treatment. Indeed, according to Childress, no medical treatment as such is obligatory; the underlying principles of beneficence and respect for persons can entail that provision of treatment is morally required, discretionary, or even wrong (1986l: 77).

Childress's position on whether there is a moral obligation to provide nutrition and hydration to patients reflects this general framework. Competent patients have a right, grounded in respect for persons, to accept or refuse insertion or implantation of a feeding tube. Proxy decision makers may likewise be morally justified in concluding that continuing medical nutrition is in the best interests of an incompetent patient. There are, however, three kinds of cases where the conditions for limited paternalism may not be satisfied.

142

First, it can be useless or futile to provide such treatment when a patient is dying and when death, no matter what actions are taken, is imminent. Medical nutrition and hydration may also be withdrawn or withheld from patients whose condition, though presumably irreversible but not imminently terminal, nevertheless rules out any possibility of benefit to the patient. Such patients include those born with anencephaly or those who are permanently unconscious or in a persistent vegetative state. In any of these situations, the provision of any medical treatment fails to meet the condition of reasonable chance of success.

Finally, when treatment may improve a patient's nutritional status, but only at great burden, particularly in the form of increased patient suffering, treatment may be considered futile in a broad sense. Provision of nutrition and hydration would then fail to meet the condition of proportionate benefit (Lynn and Childress 1983: 18-19). However, while the duty to prolong life may be justifiably infringed by decisions of either patients or proxies, the extent of infringement is limited by both beneficence and respect: refusal of medical treatment does not preclude expressions of compassion or acts of caring, such as moistening lips or massaging the body, by caregivers.

Childress's conclusions hold for a quite limited set of conditions and patients. The patient-centered approach imposes serious constraints on decision makers. Medical ambiguity, conditioned in part by our propensity for fallibility in finitude, is a key consideration in assessing the burdens and benefits of treatment, and should dispose decision makers to err (if they are to err) on the side of prolonging life. Moreover, the priority of patient interests should prevent external considerations, such as economic rationality and costs of treatment to others, from entering into, let alone controlling, the moral decision about terminating treatment.

Some difficult questions remain. It is not always clear whether Childress's argument against the provision of medical nutrition and hydration is primarily an objection to the treatment itself or to the medical technologies required to provide it, all of which involve some degree of invasiveness or constraint. This distinction may well invoke the fifth condition of limited paternalism, which requires providing benefits by the least intrusive means. In any case, his position relies on a conceptual claim that "medical procedures to provide nutrition and hydration are more similar to other medical procedures than to typical human ways of providing nutrition and hydration, for example, a sip of water" (Lynn and Childress 1983: 20-21). If so, then the underlying issue is the appropriate use of medical technology, not a recommendation about "starving" patients.

Childress's views, moreover, have undergone a noticeable evolution. Originally, he maintained that his argument did not establish an "obligation to withdraw or withhold such procedures," but only a moral permission. More recently, he has moved to a view that it can be morally obligatory not to provide artificial nutrition and hydration because it *violates* patient interests (1986l: 77-81). This stronger claim seems required by the moral logic of his argument: If the contemplated intervention fails to satisfy the necessary conditions of limited paternalism, it is not clear why the provision of treatment would be a matter of moral discretion rather than prohibition. One could affirm a discretionary stance out of respect for the interests of the patient's family (as Childress does), but this moves away from a *patient*-centered treatment standard.

Childress acknowledges that the interests of others besides the patient morally count in a decisive way. However, these others are not family members but patients in need of scarce resources that otherwise might be "wasted." Childress carefully distinguishes between decisions to forgo treatment based on the economic interests of a family or health care institution and those based on genuine claims of other patients to needed care. These latter claims, supported by the principle of justice, are particularly compelling in debates over how to allocate scarce resources.

VI. Rationing Medical Treatment

How should resources for medical care be distributed when there are more patients in need than available supplies? Childress's first foray into medical ethics addressed this question in the context of a shortage of kidney dialysis machines in the 1970s. The arguments presented in "Who Shall Live When Not All Can Live?" (1970: 339-55) remain compelling today as our society confronts scarcities of organs or drugs for AIDS patients. Childress draws upon both theological and nontheological considerations to argue that a randomizing procedure (such as queuing or a lottery) ought to be used to decide how to ration scarce, indispensable medical resources.

The ethical task, he contends, is to identify the most satisfactory criteria and procedures for determining who should live when all cannot. The selection of ethically acceptable criteria for rationing conditions the adoption of an appropriate procedure. However, the choice of criteria itself will be constrained by cultural pluralism as well as by basic convictions about human nature (1970: 342).

A first set of criteria concerns rules of exclusion that determine an initial group of medically acceptable candidates. The relevant considerations at this stage are medical need and probability of benefit, minimum standards that at least preclude wasting already scarce resources. The medical nature of these criteria determines how the procedure is implemented: health care professionals are best suited to make such judgments. Public accountability and justification by professionals are essential, however, lest medical need and benefit be expanded to encompass psychosocial considerations and assessments of the social worth of a particular patient. To guard against unjustifiable exclusion of some patients on grounds of social worth, Childress maintains that the rules of exclusion should be applied as if the scarce resource were unlimited (1981: 92; 1978: 1415).

The use of social worth criteria to determine acceptable candidates mistakenly assumes a consensus on what is valuable; the presence of pluralism argues against a selection method based on social worth. Such criteria would also require the establishment of a socially representative committee to determine who receives resources. Not only is it unlikely in theory that such a committee could adequately reflect all of society's values and determine how to rank them accurately, but in past practice, the use of "God squads" at various institutions has produced notoriously arbitrary decisions (1978: 1416; Ramsey 1970: 242-52).

Social worth judgments also reflect utilitarian assessments of past and future contributions to society. Proposing that patients receive scarce resources according to their anticipated contributions to societal well-being overlooks the dimensions of human finitude and fallibility. It is, Childress argues, "rarely easy to predict what our needs will be in a few years and what the consequences of present actions will be. Furthermore, it is difficult to predict which persons will fulfill their potential function in society. . . . We simply lack the capacity to predict very accurately the consequences which we then must evaluate. Our incapacity is never more evident than when we think in societal terms" (1970: 345-46).

There is another fundamental objection to rationing resources on grounds of social worth. A selection method that requires comparative evaluations of a mother, a minister, and an attorney, for example, reduces the value of the individual to his or her social role and function. It "dulls and perhaps even eliminates the sense of the person's transcendence, his dignity as a person" (1970: 346). The *imago Dei* here lends theological support to Childress's argument. From a theological perspective, social worth criteria simply do not adequately account for "that of God in every person."

Respect for personal dignity, Childress maintains, can best be affirmed through random selection of recipients. Whether a natural (first-come, first-served) or artificial (lottery) method is used, such a procedure maintains "a significant degree of personal dignity providing equality of opportunity" (1970: 348). Each individual has an equal right to be saved when not all can be saved.

Random selection can also sustain and extend trust, an essential aspect of human dignity (1970: 349). Patients would not be the object of interpersonal comparisons of worth by those to whom they have entrusted their care; nor would they be treated merely as means to the social good; at the same time, physicians could continue in their commitment to seek their patient's best interests without moral compromise through involvement in a selection committee.

Childress's argument for a random method is buttressed by both anthropological and theological considerations. Choosing a procedure for selecting recipients without knowing the consequences to oneself or the society of this choice both acknowledges and mitigates the factor of self-interestedness in human action. In addition, Childress reflects the views of Paul Ramsey in holding that the experience of God's indiscriminate love for human beings provides a morally significant analogy that favors equality in rationing decisions and rules out social worth assessments (1981: 94).

In our pluralistic society, Childress assumes cultural consensus on one fundamental value, equality of opportunity. This seems a plausible claim, but what is less certain is that the different methods of random selection equally guarantee equal opportunity. A natural rationing method of first-come, first-served may exclude some individuals who cannot make their need for scarce resources known soon enough because of income stratification or proximity to a medically underserved locale. Some persons may not be able to get on a waiting list for an organ transplant because they lack access to basic medical care.

An artificial method like a lottery may be morally preferable, and

146

analogically could be supported by biblical narratives. In particular, Childress points to the Jonah narrative (Jonah 1:4-7) or the selection of Matthias as one of the twelve apostles after the resurrection of Jesus (Acts 1:23-26), in which the divine will is revealed through the casting of lots: "The lot is cast into the lap; but the whole disposing thereof is of the Lord" (Proverbs 16:33). These examples again illustrate how scripture functions in Childress's ethical method to illuminate obligations.

Whether queuing or a lottery is preferable for Childress finally seems to turn on practicality. If, for example, shipwreck survivors were required to swim for a lifeboat, those who arrive first would have good grounds to dismiss calls for a lottery by those who arrive later. In this respect, Childress holds that background constraints and injustices are equally applicable to both methods. The morally critical point is that either form of randomization is preferable to an ethically unacceptable social worth approach.[5]

The scarcities that might deprive individual patients of needed or desired resources on moral grounds of fairness and equality of opportunity do not occur in isolation from much broader questions about social priorities in the allocation of health care resources. Macroallocation issues — how much a society spends on health care relative to other social goods; how it divides health expenditures among preventive, chronic, and acute care medicine; how it assigns priorities to different diseases and technologies — all affect the amount of individual resources to be distributed among individual patients, and thus can determine the extent of the problem of scarcity (1979b: 256-69). For example, some state legislatures recently have limited funds for organ transplants in order to enhance prenatal care programs. A limited supply of organs for transplant not only creates perplexing choices at the microdecision level (which patient should receive an available organ), but also poses important questions about society's policy alternatives (1987b: 85-110).

5. Childress does allow exceptions "in some emergency situations" for social utility concerns to take precedence, based on "specific, urgent functions" a person or group might perform for the common good (1983b: 551-54, 561). For example, a leader of a country might be given treatment priority to ensure societal survival.

VII. "Gifts of Life": Organ Procurement

In distributing the scarce resource of transplantable organs, Childress would follow the general criteria of fair rationing described above, though in his participation as vice-chair of the National Task Force on Organ Transplantation, he has viewed the queuing approach as a more efficient method of distribution. Yet it must be acknowledged that this shortage is at least theoretically avoidable. Estimates indicate there are more than enough deaths each year in the U.S. to provide "a surfeit of organs" (1986b: 133). Childress has thus also devoted considerable attention to identifying a morally acceptable method of organ procurement that would effectively alleviate shortages when implemented.

He agrees with many that the predominant procurement method of the last two decades, encouraging voluntary gifts of organs through public education and distribution of donor cards, has simply failed to furnish a sufficient number of suitable organs. While Childress holds that a variety of policies — including express or presumed donation or commercial sales — may be ethically permissible, the challenge for policymakers is to identify morally preferable and politically feasible alternatives (1989b: 89).

Because social priorities and public policy loom large in the consideration of procurement alternatives, Childress's own ethical and policy conclusions are justified by nontheological reasoning. He has nevertheless sought to discern the implications of basic themes in Western religious traditions, such as the *imago Dei* and *agape*, embodiment and stewardship, for individual and family decisions about donation. This is a significant consideration as religious beliefs may contribute to the general scarcity of organs. Opinion surveys reveal that people's reluctance to donate organs stems from concern about the integrity of the body in the "resurrection or afterlife" among 12 percent of respondents and from "religious prohibitions" in 9 percent (Report 1986: 37-39, 142). Such beliefs are not as central in creating shortages as is pervasive distrust of health care institutions, but questions can be raised about the relation of religious convictions and societal procurement methods.

The *imago Dei* presents a particularly important theme for thinking about organ donation within a religious context, since it supports a concept of human stewardship over creation and over the use and disposal of one's body and body parts. "As stewards and trustees, human beings do not have unlimited power. God has set limits on what human

148

beings may do with and to their own bodies and the bodies of others" (1989a: 218). The model of stewardship imposes obligations toward the body, living or dead, especially respect for the cadaver; demands justification for invasions of the body, including for purposes of organ procurement; and establishes a presumption in favor of respecting the wishes of persons regarding organ donation (1989a: 230).

The current procurement system, moreover, is structured by the model and language of "gifts" and is characterized by Childress as "encouraged altruism." In organ donation, "gifts of life" are typically offered to unknown, unidentified strangers in critical need. Such a model is not incompatible with religious perspectives concerning the body's sanctity and the requirement for justification. For example, Childress notes that the strong prohibitions in Jewish traditions against desecration of the corpse, rooted in the *imago Dei*, like "any prohibition in Jewish law, except for murder, incest and idolatry, may be overridden in order to save human life" (1989a: 220). Moreover, procurement methods structured by the notions of altruism, gift, and generosity may provide an occasion for the expression of *agape* and concern for the neighbor's welfare. "It may be an act of love to donate one's organs before or after death, or a deceased relative's organs, in order to meet a neighbor's needs" (1986h: 441). Within a religious community, the more closely procurement policies conform to a gift model, the less likely they seem to risk infringing the boundaries of the *imago Dei*.

Whether seeing the decision about organ donation as a discretionary gift will solve the *social* problem of shortages is another question. Childress clearly thinks not, and has recently affirmed that, at least with respect to the donation of kidneys, "both individuals and their family members have an obligation of beneficence to donate cadaver organs to benefit patients suffering from end-stage organ failure" (Beauchamp and Childress 1989: 207). Nevertheless, societal procurement efforts are constrained by the principle of respect for persons, including respect for their religious convictions. Such respect precludes "expropriation" policies in which cadaver organs would be retrieved irrespective of or even against the expressed wishes of the decedent. The *imago Dei* and stewardship concepts would provide religious reasons to reject such an alternative because of its implicit disrespect for the cadaver. Moreover, expropriation is contrary to the altruism that supports current practices and may even be counterproductive over time by heightening distrust (such as fears over premature declaration of death) about the procurement system and the lengths it will go to save the lives of others. Though expropriation may theoretically be a very efficient way to increase the supply of organs, moral, theological, and political objections exclude it as a viable policy option (1989b: 98-99).

Commercial sales of transplantable organs may be ethically acceptable, based on respect for a donor's freedom of choice, although there are moral concerns about the voluntariness of the choice and the potential for exploitation in a market system where demand is great. However, Childress does not view an "organ market" as significantly more effective in increasing the supply of organs. Nor would such a method express altruism or support the practice of gift-giving. The *imago Dei* and stewardship themes likewise support reluctance to endorse this policy option, for a commercial market in organs may encourage viewing human bodies and their parts as commodities. For several reasons, then, Childress contends, "It would be ethically and politically unwise to convert the system of donation into a system of sales until [alternative] policies have been given a chance to work, in part because transfer of organs by sales would be costly, would probably drive out many donations, and could have serious effects on our conception of personhood and embodiment by promoting commodification (1989b: 101-2).

A policy based on "presumed consent" to organ donation is held by Childress to be ethically permissible to the extent that personal choices are the controlling factor (1986b: 138). However, it is subject to scrutiny at several points. The element of consent may be substantially diminished if organs are removed routinely from cadavers only because donors do not dissent. The failure to dissent cannot automatically be construed as consent; silence may instead indicate that donors do not know about or understand the procurement process.

While Childress believes that "a policy of presumed donation rests on passive altruism, and it does not preclude active altruism," he also contends that "a policy of express consent is ethically preferable, because it promotes active generosity and community" (1986h: 442). The difficult tension for Childress is how he can reconcile his evident interest in perpetuating a "gift" model of organ donation with the claim that such donation is an obligation of beneficence, since we ordinarily do not conceive of altruistic acts as obligatory. Moreover, the moral priority of express consent, it has already been indicated, has historically been an inefficient method for obtaining organs.

These somewhat divergent objectives, Childress believes, may best be balanced by the policy alternative of "required request," in which the key element is the development of "institutional [e.g., hospital] protocols for approaching the family of a dead person who is a potential source of organs" (1989b: 94). Health care professionals may ask family members about the wishes of the decedent with respect to organ donation and, if these are unknown, could inform the family of their moral and legal right to donate. Moreover, this approach allows the family to exercise "responsive generosity or charity." And while in some instances this may entail moving the locus of consent from the individual to the family, Childress contends that "it is appropriate to view the family as entrusted with the corpse and thus as stewards and trustees, who should act on the decedent's wishes where they are known, but who may make their own decisions about donation if the decedent's wishes are not known" (1989a: 233). In this respect, Childress believes that his advocacy of express consent and required request as preferred and feasible organ procurement policies can be harmonized with the ethical and theological significance of gifts, stewardship, and respect for the body as a symbol of the image of God.

VIII. Ethics and Policy:
The Community of Ethical Responsibility

Childress has called for more careful analytical and constructive attention to the moral norms — such as love and justice — that are invoked in bioethics discourse as a means to clarify and resolve some controversial issues, while acknowledging "the impossibility of either clarifying or resolving these disputes without attention to [the] broader theological, metaphysical and anthropological contexts" of such norms (1985: 225). I have tried to indicate how these broader premoral presuppositions inform Childress's own ethical method, and how this method can assist decision makers confronting perplexing bioethics issues. Still, we might ask Childress to heed his own call and articulate his own constructive position in certain areas.

Childress's appeal to "discernment" and "prudence" to determine the morally fitting principle for a situation, for example, looks suspiciously like reliance on intuitionism. This limitation is made even more serious by his moral anthropology. If finitude, fallibility, and sin infect moral decision making to the extent Childress claims, the capacity of persons to discern the winning principle in cases of conflict would seem similarly suspect. Philosophers and theologians since Aristotle and Aquinas have warned against expecting undue precision in ethics, acknowledging that uncertainty increases the more concrete ethics becomes. Nevertheless, absent what both Aristotle and Aquinas provided, an account of discernment and prudence in moral reasoning, it is not clear that Childress's method provides solid grounds for any decision made in a situation where two principles conflict.

One possible remedy is the articulation of a theory of value, particularly regarding the substantive goods that constitute human flourishing and well-being. Childress's interpretation of the "nature" of human beings is in my view existentially and theologically insightful and realistic. But we are told very little about the "destiny" of human beings — the goods toward which we are naturally inclined or that we ought to be pursuing. Perhaps finitude and fallibility inhibit or prevent apprehension of ultimate human ends; but the central challenge that developing a concept of human destiny may pose for Childress's ethics is whether it is possible to articulate a substantive account of human well-being without risking the imperialism of paternalism.

The concern about human destiny and meaning has been central for theological traditions and religious communities. One clear implication of Childress's view that the meaning and weight of moral norms is connected with deeper metaphysical convictions is that the theological claims of particular communities can alter the moral meaning and significance of principles such as love of neighbor or respect for persons. In this regard, attention to the moral discourse of distinctive theological traditions or, more generally, particular cultures may suggest limits to the scope of Childress's method, relying as it does on a "common morality."

This point notwithstanding, a tradition-bound medical ethics risks silencing theological perspectives in the moral discourse of the public realm and ensures that the responsibility for fashioning ethically sound health policies will be undertaken without the leaven of religious insights. Childress's ethics indicates the need for accountability, for *theological* reasons, to claims and interests beyond those of particular religious communities. Consistent with this, he has been an active participant, as both specialist and citizen, in several national commissions charged with making specific public policy recommendations on difficult ethical issues, such as organ transplantation, human gene therapy, and fetal tissue transplantation (1991). The ethicist is indeed directed and called to reflect on social and policy concerns out of the responsibility of "answering . . . every person." In this very fundamental mode of engagement with rather than withdrawal from vexing policy issues, theological convictions may have their most profound impact on the dilemmas of medical ethics.

References

Beauchamp, Tom L., and James F. Childress. 1989. *Principles of Biomedical Ethics,* 3d ed. New York: Oxford University Press.

Butler, Joseph. 1983. "A Dissertation Upon the Nature of Virtue." In *Five Sermons,* ed. Stephen L. Darwall. Indianapolis: Hackett.

Childress, James F. 1970. "Who Shall Live When Not All Can Live?" *Soundings* 53, no. 4: 339-55.

―――. 1971. *Civil Disobedience and Political Obligation: A Study in Christian Social Ethics.* New Haven: Yale University Press.

―――. 1974. "'Answering That of God in Every Man' — An Interpretation of George Fox's Ethics." *Quaker Religious Thought* 15: 2-41.

―――. 1978. "Rationing of Medical Treatment." In *Encyclopedia of Bioethics,* ed. Warren T. Reich. New York: Free Press.

―――. 1979a. "Appeals to Conscience." *Ethics* 89: 315-35.

―――. 1979b. "Priorities in the Allocation of Health Care Resources." *Soundings* 62, no. 3: 256-74.

―――. 1980. "Paternalism and Autonomy in Medical Decision-Making." In *Frontiers in Medical Ethics: Applications in a Medical Setting,* ed. Virginia Abernethy, 27-41. Cambridge, Mass.: Ballinger.

―――. 1981. *Priorities in Biomedical Ethics.* Philadelphia: Westminster Press.

―――. 1982a. "Metaphors and Models of Medical Relationships." In *Social Responsibility: Journalism, Law and Medicine,* ed. Louis Hodges, 47-70. Lexington, Va.: Washington and Lee University Press.

―――. 1982b. *Moral Responsibility in Conflicts: Essays on Nonviolence, War and Conscience.* Baton Rouge: Louisiana State University Press.

―――. 1982c. *Who Should Decide? Paternalism in Health Care.* New York: Oxford University Press.

―――. 1983a. "Scripture and Christian Ethics: Some Reflections on the Role of Scripture in Moral Deliberation and Justification." In *Readings in Moral Theology, No. 4: The Use of Scripture in Moral Theology,* ed. Charles E. Curran and Richard A. McCormick, 276-88. Ramsey, N.H.: Paulist Press.

————. 1983b. "Triage in Neonatal Intensive Care: The Limitations of a Metaphor." *Virginia Law Review* 69, no. 3: 547-610.

————. 1984a. "Ensuring Care, Respect and Fairness for the Elderly." *Hastings Center Report* 14, no. 5: 27-31.

————. 1984b. "Rights to Health Care in a Democratic Society." In *Biomedical Ethics Reviews,* ed. Robert Almeder and James Humber, 47-70. Clifton, N.J.: Humana Press.

————. 1985. "Love and Justice in Christian Biomedical Ethics." In *Theology and Bioethics: Exploring the Foundations and Frontiers,* ed. Earl E. Shelp, 225-43. Boston: D. Reidel.

————. 1986a. "Autonomy." In *The Westminster Dictionary of Christian Ethics,* ed. James F. Childress and John Macquarrie. Philadelphia: Westminster Press.

————. 1986b. "The Gift of Life: Ethical Problems and Policies in Obtaining and Distributing Organs for Transplantation." *Critical Care Clinics* 2, no. 1: 133-48.

————. 1986c. "Image of God *(Imago Dei)*." In *The Westminster Dictionary of Christian Ethics,* ed. James F. Childress and John Macquarrie. Philadelphia: Westminster Press.

————. 1986d. "Justification, Moral." In *The Westminster Dictionary of Christian Ethics,* ed. James F. Childress and John Macquarrie. Philadelphia: Westminster Press.

————. 1986e. "The Meaning of the 'Right to Life'." In *Natural Rights and Natural Law: The Legacy of George Mason,* ed. Robert P. Davidson, 123-67. Fairfax, Va.: George Mason University Press.

————. 1986f. "Nonmaleficence." In *The Westminster Dictionary of Christian Ethics,* ed. James F. Childress and John Macquarrie. Philadelphia: Westminster Press.

————. 1986g. "Norms." In *The Westminster Dictionary of Christian Ethics,* ed. James F. Childress and John Macquarrie. Philadelphia: Westminster Press.

————. 1986h. "Organ Transplantation." In *The Westminster Dictionary of Christian Ethics,* ed. James F. Childress and John Macquarrie. Philadelphia: Westminster Press.

————. 1986i. "Paternalism." In *The Westminster Dictionary of Christian Ethics,* ed. James F. Childress and John Macquarrie. Philadelphia: Westminster Press.

————. 1986j. "Proportionality, Principle of." In *The Westminster Dictionary of Christian Ethics,* ed. James F. Childress and John Macquarrie. Philadelphia: Westminster Press.

————. 1986k. "Situation Ethics." In *The Westminster Dictionary of Christian Ethics,* ed. James F. Childress and John Macquarrie. Philadelphia: Westminster Press.

————. 1986l. "When Is It Morally Justifiable to Discontinue Medical Nutri-
tion and Hydration?" In *By No Extraordinary Means: The Choice to Forgo
Life-Sustaining Food and Water,* ed. Joanne Lynn, 67-83. Bloomington:
Indiana University Press.

————. 1987a. "An Ethical Framework for Assessing Policies to Screen for
Antibodies to HIV." *AIDS and Public Policy Journal* 2 (Winter): 28-31.

————. 1987b. "Some Moral Connections Between Organ Procurement and
Organ Distribution." *Journal of Contemporary Health Law and Policy* 3:
85-110.

————. 1989a. "Attitudes of Major Western Religious Traditions toward Uses
of the Human Body and Its Parts." In *Justice and The Holy: Essays in
Honor of Walter Harrelson,* ed. Douglas A. Knight and Peter J. Paris,
215-40. Atlanta: Scholars Press.

————. 1989b. "Ethical Criteria for Procuring and Distributing Organs for
Transplantation." *Journal of Health Politics, Policy and Law* 14: 87-113.

————. 1989c. "The Normative Principles of Medical Ethics." In *Medical
Ethics,* ed. Robert M. Veatch, 28-47. Boston: Jones and Bartlett.

————. 1990a. "Dissassociation from Evil: The Case of Human Fetal Tissue
Transplantation Research." In *Social Responsibility: Business, Journalism,
Law, Medicine,* ed. Louis W. Hodges, 32-49. Lexington, Va.: Washington
and Lee University Press.

————. 1990b. "The Place of Autonomy in Bioethics." *Hastings Center Report*
20, no. 1: 12-17.

————. 1991. "Ethics, Public Policy, and Human Fetal Tissue Transplantation."
Kennedy Institute of Ethics Journal 1, no. 2: 93-121.

Childress, James F., and Courtney S. Campbell. 1989. " 'Who Is a Doctor to
Decide Whether a Person Lives or Dies?': Reflections on Dax's Case." In
Dax's Case: Essays in Medical Ethics and Human Meaning, ed. Lonnie D.
Kliever, 23-41. Dallas: Southern Methodist University Press.

Childress, James F., and Mark Siegler. 1984. "Metaphors and Models of Doc-
tor-Patient Relationships: Their Implications for Autonomy." *Theoretical
Medicine* 5: 17-30.

Gustafson, James M. 1978. "Theology Confronts Technology and the Life Sciences." *Commonweal* 105: 386-92.

Jonas, Hans. 1984. *The Imperative of Responsibility: In Search of an Ethics for
the Technological Age.* Chicago: University of Chicago Press.

Kant, Immanuel. 1969. *Foundations of the Metaphysics of Morals,* trans. Lewis
White Beck. Indianapolis: Bobbs-Merrill.

Lynn, Joanne, and James F. Childress. 1983. "Must Patients Always Be Given
Food and Water?" *Hastings Center Report* 13, no. 5: 17-21.

Niebuhr, H. Richard. 1942. "War as the Judgment of God." *Christian Century*
59: 630-33.

————. 1963. *The Responsible Self: An Essay in Christian Moral Philosophy.* San Francisco: Harper and Row.

Niebuhr, Reinhold. 1964. *The Nature and Destiny of Man.* New York: Charles Scribner's Sons.

Ramsey, Paul. 1970. *The Patient as Person.* New Haven: Yale University Press.

Report of the Task Force on Organ Transplantation. 1986. *Organ Transplantation: Issues and Recommendations.* Washington, D.C.: U.S. Department of Health and Human Services.

Smith, David H. 1987. "On Paul Ramsey: A Covenant-Centered Ethic for Medicine." *Second Opinion* 6 (November): 106-27.

Weber, Max. 1958. "Politics as a Vocation." In *From Max Weber: Essays in Sociology,* ed. H. H. Gerth and C. Wright Mills, 77-128. New York: Oxford University Press.

ON GERMAIN GRISEZ

Can Christian Ethics Give Answers?

JAMES G. HANINK

Critical Times and Hard Questions

A GOOD many people see this century as a time of protracted moral crisis. Even the eruption of democracy in Eastern Europe and the promising redirection of the republics of the former Soviet Union take place against the backdrop of widespread misgivings about "the end of nature" and humanity's abuse of creation. There are crises enough to give most of us frequent occasion to doubt our judgments and to re-explore our intellectual and moral traditions. Questions of medical ethics especially provide such occasions.

Christian thinkers are scarcely immune to doubt. But faith, they maintain, makes a critical difference. Reflective Christians should be ready to explore, with measured confidence, the crises that we all face. Even nonbelievers should welcome such an enterprise. If nothing else, it will provide them with a "second opinion" on a whole range of disputed questions, and worthy colleagues in an ongoing public conversation.

It is this readiness to address the hard questions, and to do so with a sturdy confidence in Christian reflection, that characterizes the work of Germain Grisez.

Grisez is a past president of the American Catholic Philosophical Association. He currently holds the Flynn Chair of Christian Ethics at Mount Saint Mary's College in Emmitsburg, Maryland, teaching moral theology and serving the single largest Roman Catholic seminary in the United States. Yet Grisez did not begin his professional life as a moral theologian. He did his graduate work in philosophy at the University of Chicago, taking his Ph.D. under the direction of the distinguished Aristotle scholar Richard McKeon. The Catholic intellectual tradition has always nourished a productive cross-fertilization between theology and philosophy. In Grisez's case, this pattern has produced a theologian with impressive analytic rigor and, at the same time, a philosopher who draws creatively on a Christian sensibility.

Germain Grisez has for years addressed a whole range of issues centering on the dignity and worth of human life. He has authored or coauthored separate volumes on contraception (1964), abortion (1970a), euthanasia (1979), and, most recently, nuclear deterrence (1987a). In the course of tackling this agenda of ethical problems — each with major public policy implications — Grisez has also developed and refined what is surely the most widely debated contemporary version of natural law moral theory. The sharpest articulation of his position appears in the long foundational essay "Practical Principles, Moral Truth, and Ultimate Ends" (1987b), coauthored with Joseph Boyle and John Finnis. Perhaps the key feature of Grisez's natural law theory is the role played by basic human goods in fulfilling human potential.

Grisez pursues a unified course, that of constructing a consistent prolife ethics that repudiates capital punishment, calls for unilateral nuclear disarmament, rejects the killing of critically ill patients, and advocates returning legal protection to fetuses. Grisez's early essay "Toward a Consistent Natural Law Ethics of Killing" (1970b) set the controversial course that he has followed for the past twenty years.

It is not easy to determine how influential Germain Grisez has been, within either the Catholic or the larger community. In the first place, philosophers and theologians are (or should be) concerned more with truth than with influence. Second, the dialectic of philosophical and theological debate is open-ended, so influence is always in flux. Nonetheless, one simply cannot understand much of the contemporary debate within the Catholic community without coming to terms with Grisez's natural law vision. One test of its impact will be the extent to which its categories appear in Pope John Paul II's anticipated new encyclical on moral principles.

Outside Catholicism, Grisez's work is now widely anthologized in academic publications. But perhaps more important, it is a respected resource for interfaith prolife activists now participating in our profound national reassessment of abortion and euthanasia.

But the hard work of coming to intellectual terms with a systematic thinker is only just begun with a thumbnail biographical sketch and a précis of thematic concerns. What we most need is a broad avenue — better yet, a network of such avenues — that helps us make contact with Germain Grisez's system and vision. Perhaps the most helpful points of contact are what we might call "questions overheard."

Most of us, however long it has been since we have done any formal work in ethics or whether we've done any at all, have participated in or overheard discussions that are tagged with questions of enduring, often problematic, moral significance. I would like to list seven such questions. For reflective adults, and perhaps especially for medical professionals, they are both familiar and disconcerting: familiar because the logic of moral inquiry forces us to raise them; disconcerting because so often we are unsure how to answer them, yet so much depends on our answers.

Seven Disconcerting Questions

Let's turn, then, to this battery of exploratory questions. In each instance I will briefly situate the question in a plausible context.

1. In the course of a friendly exchange, three medical professionals — X, Y, and Z — first clarify the difference between factual claims ("the patient suffers from AIDS") and moral claims ("the patient ought to have access to an experimental drug"). Soon their discussion moves from analysis to advocacy. X insists that the drug should be provided; Y claims the opposite. Puzzled, the more skeptical Z asks, "In making moral judgments, can anyone claim to *know*? Maybe we can only express our feelings."

2. The adult daughter of an elderly, infirm patient has been tragically killed in a boating accident. Should the patient be told? The patient's spouse says, "He'll only be upset." The patient's son disagrees. "He has a right to know. No one is really happy being deceived." A nurse silently muses, "What's happiness, anyway?"

3. "I'm against abandoning sick people, period," says a hospital administrator about to bring suit against a Christian Science couple

who refuse to allow their daughter any further treatment other than prayer. "But we don't want your kind of care," the couple responds. A judge who hears the case knows what the law requires but, off the record, asks a colleague, "Are there universal moral truths? Or are there 'cultural breaks' at work?"

4. A physician visiting a cancer hospice finds himself listening to a fervent request for euthanasia. He answers, "I never kill my patients. That is a basic principle." Hearing of the request, one of the physician's partners asks herself, "Are there really moral absolutes?"

5. A medical intern discovers she has a strong interest in and talent for obstetrics. She is offered a position in a major hospital where, from time to time, abortions are performed. Would she be willing to perform them? In another hospital, a resident is invited to join a team that will "harvest" organs from anencephalic babies who have been maintained on life support systems. Each young physician raises a fundamental question. The first asks, "When does human life really begin?" The second asks, "When does human life really end?"

6. A committee of beleaguered hospital administrators has spent a week lobbying its county board of supervisors to allocate more funds for trauma centers. It has not been easy going, since even the most sympathetic supervisors have emphasized that the county's resources are sharply limited and that there are other urgent needs. One of the administrators asks a colleague, "What amount of our public resources ought we direct to health care?" Testily, the colleague counters, "How much is a human life worth?"

7. Surprisingly, a poll of a regional nurses' association shows that a majority of its members oppose abortion on demand. A meeting of the association's executive board raises the question, Should the association support legal restrictions on abortion? In discussion, one puzzled nurse asks, "What role should the law play in mandating morality?"

Seven scenarios, seven "questions overheard." Germain Grisez's work suggests a way of answering each. In keeping with Grisez's Christian natural law perspective, the answers grow out of rational reflection on our shared experience of human nature. At this point we are in position to begin outlining Grisez's moral philosophy and indicating the theological resources on which it draws. Only when we have done so can we return to our seven questions with integrated answers for our consideration.

A Christian Natural Law Ethics

A moral philosophy within the natural law tradition sees actions as right insofar as they help to realize the full potential of human nature and wrong insofar as they frustrate the full realization of that potential. But so general a definition tells us little unless we know something of the historical background of the natural law vision; understand what a natural law thinker like Grisez takes human nature to be; and work through the account of values or basic goods that he proposes. Only when we have accomplished this can we clearly state Germain Grisez's fundamental moral standard and, finally, see how his system of ethics converges with pivotal Christian beliefs.

Our first task, then, is to point to some historical antecedents of Grisez's thought. He has borrowed widely and constructively.[1]

From Socrates, Grisez accepts the view that there are moral truths, that they do not depend simply on one's culture, and that reason can at least sometimes recognize these truths. Socrates, for example, taught that an examined life is ethically richer than an unexamined one, whether in Athens, Sparta, or Persia. One of the implications of this is that we can claim a measure of moral confidence. Genocide is wrong, and we know it. Though often we state moral truths with great feeling, these truths are not reducible to our feelings. Another implication is that moral truth is not culturally restricted, anymore than antibiotics are. Racism, for example, is wrong everywhere.

From Aristotle, Grisez brings us the conviction not only that the task of ethics is showing us how to realize our potential but that we can realize that potential only in communities. The implication is that moral questions characteristically have social answers. This is a difficult lesson for American individualism to master, but we pay a heavy price for our obduracy.

From Aquinas, Grisez brings as an ideal not the rigid separation of faith and ethics but their mutual support. The overarching implication of this ideal is that we need never be apologetic in supposing that Christian faith contributes positively to ethical analysis. Though theology must be critical if ethical analysis is to succeed, it cannot close itself off from the transcendent.

---

1. For an attempt to link Grisez's Thomistic natural law theory with the divine command ethics of the Reformed tradition, see Hanink and Mar 1987.

From the Enlightenment period, Grisez recovers an emphasis on the rights of the person. A critical implication of this is that the common good ought never exclude the good of even a single person. Christianity offers a transcendent horizon to this conviction. Thus Grisez recalls Aquinas's thesis that "human persons are not ordered to political society according to all they are and have, but rather to God," and notes that faith "teaches that subordination to divine goodness requires not the destruction of persons but their fulfillment" (1983: 273). Persons are never expendable. We will see that Grisez strengthens the foundation of this thesis.

An understanding of human nature, whatever its historical debts, must stand on its own. If ethics is about realizing the full potential of human nature, how is it that Grisez understands that nature? And what does he see as its distinctive goods?

Sometimes we best can understand an account of the human person by contrasting it with sharply competing views. A utilitarian like John Stuart Mill sees human nature as most sharply characterized by a seeking of pleasure and an avoiding of pain. A critical rationalist like Immanuel Kant emphasizes the sovereign place of reason. Social contract thinkers like Thomas Hobbes call attention to the driving force of enlightened self-interest.

Grisez sees a different dynamic as far more central to human nature. Neither hedonist, rationalist, nor contractarian, Grisez calls our attention to the special place of reflective freedom. We humans are deeply affected by our biological and cultural endowments. But we are nonetheless free agents. As such we characteristically can choose both our actions' ends and the means to realize them. Beyond this, we can reflect on our freedom and its purposiveness. Indeed, we can cooperate with one another to promote more fully this goal-oriented freedom.

For Grisez, the human capacity for reflective freedom helps us understand why scripture teaches us that we are fashioned in God's very image (Genesis 1:26-27). But this priceless freedom comes into its own only when we work to realize the whole range of basic goods open to us. In turning to these goods, we move to the distinctive core of Grisez's natural law ethics, his axiology.

The first point to make about the basic goods is that we human beings do indeed find them attractive. Far from being distractions or obstacles, our natural inclinations point us to the basic goods. But just what are these goods — the states of affairs, to use the broadest heading, to which we are nearly all attracted? Grisez would include at least the following: life, knowledge, aesthetic appreciation, friendship (of which sexual community is a distinctive form), excellence in work or play, self-integration, authenticity, and holiness.

Each of these goods, moreover, is in its own way a dimension of the person. Friendship, for example, is not some entity distinct from the friends who share in it. Rather, it is an aspect of their very persons. Nor is knowledge something external to us. Rather, it is lived; it is an aspect of the person who knows. As dimensions of people, basic goods have an intrinsic rather than merely instrumental worth. Moreover, while one sometimes can buy the means to a basic good, such goods themselves cannot be bought.

For Grisez, each of the basic goods is a constituent of human flourishing or integral fulfillment. This fulfillment is, to use the classical term, our *telos*. Our unifying goal in life is not merely realizing our potential in a limited role, skill, or function. We aim instead to develop a kind of human excellence.

But why, a skeptic might persist, is this development itself good? For Grisez, the answer lies in God's creative wisdom. "While in God there can be no distinction between what he is and what he ought to be, each creature has a role in the order of things which it ought to fulfill. Its fulfillment and fullness of being will be that share in the expression of the divine goodness which God intended for it in creating it" (1983: 118). Thus Grisez anchors human goodness in the very structure of God's creation. Given this foundation, he can observe that "since human goodness is found in the fullness of human being, one begins to understand what it is to be a good person by considering what things fulfill human persons. Things which do so are human goods in the central sense . . . [and] aspects of persons, not realities apart from persons" (1983: 121). But integral fulfillment, our realizing of the basic goods that are the building blocks of our flourishing as *humans* (rather than, say, as citizens, medical professionals, or academics), does not automatically result from following our inclinations. Reason must direct our free responses to the basic goods. Reason directs us to pursue them in a coherent way and never attack or demean them, whether we are focusing on ourselves or on others.

Nonetheless, since we recognize a plurality of goods, it is clear that one cannot equally pursue them all. Indeed, one cannot equally pursue all instances of a particular good. Consider, for example, the medical researcher who is devoted to the already specific good of medical science. She cannot be equally expert in every area of contemporary medicine, much less in every area of medicine plus art history at the same time.

Since our human limitations prevent us from equally pursuing and realizing all the basic goods, how should we proceed? Might we, for example, use one good to negotiate for another? Can we use them as bargaining chips?

Here Grisez makes a striking claim about the basic goods. They are both incommensurable and nonfungible. That is, they admit of no common measure enabling us to say that one is more valuable than another. Nor without loss could we replace one basic good with another, or even with another instance of the same sort of good.

A pair of examples illustrates these concepts. The first example is extreme, though a good many philosophers have speculated about it. Suppose, because of a shortage of cadaver organs, we could save five persons only by "harvesting" the vital organs of one. Incommensurability insists that we cannot justify the killing of one to save five because we cannot commensurate the value of life. Nor could we save five friendships by betraying a legitimate trust that would destroy another relationship; life and friendship are both incommensurable goods.

The second example, illustrating what it is for a good to be nonfungible, is only too familiar to obstetrical nurses and physicians. A mother loses a baby, perhaps her first. A well-meaning friend says, "It's hard. But everything will be all right . . . you'll have another." Commodities, like bushels of soybeans, are fungible — exchangeable. Babies are not. Nor are friendships or any other of the basic goods.

With respect to the basic good of life, at least, Grisez's uncompromising position is one that the late Paul Ramsey shared. Grisez, moreover, shares Ramsey's sobering view of just how much is at stake: "The notion that an individual human life is absolutely unique, inviolable, irreplaceable, noninterchangeable, not substitutable, and not meldable with other lives is a notion that exists in our civilization because it is Christian; and that idea is so fundamental in the edifice of Western law and morals that it cannot be removed without bringing the whole house down" (1978: xiv).

A further point Grisez is especially anxious to underscore is that the morality of an action is not simply a function of its external effects. Choice is not just a means to bring about some external state of affairs. Rather, moral choice is equally "concerned with the fulfillment of persons in their existential dimensions — a fulfillment which resides mainly in individual and communal choices, not in definite states of affairs which result from carrying them out" (1983: 161). When we reflect on actions as transforming their agents, a merely consequentialist calculus seems doubly suspect, first, because there is no objective scale for ranking various envisioned sets of external consequences; second, because such a calculus largely overlooks the developing character of the agent — a character that is constructed by the choices the agent makes.

Yet how are we to proceed, given a plurality of incommensurable and nonfungible basic goods? Is Grisez's panoply of basic goods perhaps too rich? In cases in which not all goods are realizable, the moral course — that is, the fully rational course — is to remain open to all of the goods and to cooperate with others so that the community, if not the individual, can realize their fullest range. (This fullest range of goods, together with their material and cultural preconditions, is what the natural law tradition has in mind when it speaks of the common good.) An illustration of this stance is that extraordinarily complex and — mostly — functional institution, the contemporary hospital. Different participants in the institution pursue different goods; yet insofar as there is genuine cooperation, the hospital community can come closer and closer to realizing the health of those it serves and the specialized knowledge needed to do so.

We have seen enough now of Grisez's understanding of the basic goods to have sketched out his axiology, or account of moral values. Consequently we can turn to what we might call his fundamental moral standard or, more informally, his "ethical bottom line." It is simply this: an action is morally right if and only if it reasonably promotes some basic good and does not, in so doing, intentionally attack another such good. The moral life is both positive and negative, both a matter of acting and of refraining. Life involves saying both "yes" and "no." This standard Grisez himself formally states in terms of ethical integration. "In voluntarily acting for human goods and avoiding what is opposed to them, one ought to choose and otherwise will those and only those possibilities whose willing is compatible with a will toward integral human fulfillment" (1983: 184).

The idea of intentionality is critical to Grisez's fundamental moral standard. While some ethicists look chiefly or exclusively to the results of our acts, Grisez would insist that what we do cannot be separated from some reference to intention. (What is the difference between, say, waving to a friend and making a hand signal for a right turn? Or what distinguishes suicide from martyrdom, since each foresees a certain death [1979: 407-12]?) Moreover, the larger moral significance of an act turns on the agent's intention. Indeed, my character is a function of the intentions with which I act.

Here a philosopher might say that the core exposition of Grisez's natural law ethics is complete. But Grisez is as much a moral theologian as a philosopher. He is not a compartmentalized thinker; certainly he does not erect a barrier between thinking as a philosopher and thinking as a Christian. I want, then, to point to the relation he sees between ethics and faith and suggest where he finds them converging.

He would say, first, that natural law ethics is autonomous. It is coherent and instructive apart from any theological reference. Still, the Catholic natural law tradition that he both draws upon and extends also argues that natural law ethics is greatly strengthened if developed in a scriptural context. Reading even a page or two of St. Thomas Aquinas shows the interplay of philosophy and scriptural reflection.

We can see this deepening of vision on both a broad epistemic and a more particular axiological level. Epistemically, it is notoriously hard to think clearly or consistently when one's own subjectivity is at issue, as it so decidedly is in ethical inquiry. But revelation and the faith tradition which give us scripture underscore and clarify what reason often only obscurely concludes.

Examples of how the vision of faith can deepen our axiology of the basic goods are both handy and provocative. The natural law thinker recognizes our appetite for life and inclination to preserve it. Yet when we see the harrowing pain that sometimes attends a life, we may begin to doubt that life is a basic good. But if, at a still deeper level, we see in faith that human life is made in God's image, then our judgment that it is such a good is reaffirmed.

Or again: there is a great difference between a purely secular analysis of "reproductive ethics" and a religiously articulate reflection on the "ethics of procreation." Both are important. But the first necessarily lacks the sacral horizon normative for the second. Only the second sees the transmission of life as sharing in God's creative action.

Or consider friendship and its distinctive expression in sexual community. From a secular perspective they are already great goods. But if we see both in the context of God's passionate covenant with

Israel, their significance in human flourishing becomes still more striking. It reaches out to the sacred.

Indeed, Grisez notes that all our moral insights are deepened by our covenant relationship with God. At the same time, that covenant gives us a fresh perspective for criticizing merely conventional morality. The prophets illustrate the latter, while Yahweh's proclamation of a new world order to Noah (Genesis 9) highlights the former.

Finally, we should see humanity's struggle to flourish in the context of creation's revelation of God's grandeur. And, amazingly, because of Christ's death and resurrection, we can go beyond a natural excellence to a share in God's own life. The struggle for the goods of human nature leads to our personal transformation in the kingdom of God. Thus grace builds on nature and, in so doing, transforms it and heals its brokenness.

Here, perhaps, a sympathetic reader might be thinking, "I now see the broad contours of this kind of ethics. I appreciate how it draws on Christian sources. But I'm still wondering about those 'questions overheard.' They won't be left hanging, will they? Put this system to work and get them answered for me!"

So let's address our original series of seven inquiries.

The first, prompted by a disagreement over whether an AIDS patient ought to have access to an experimental drug was: "When making moral judgments, can anyone claim to know?" Against the several forms of noncognitivism, Grisez would answer that there are moral truths and that sometimes we can know them. Reflection on our experience enables us to recognize the basic goods, and natural law tells us that we are to pursue them. The more specific and context-dependent the judgment is, the more circumspect we must be in our knowledge claims. But if, for example, someone charged with war crimes were to protest, "But I didn't know that it was wrong to torture and kill noncombatants," we simply would dismiss the excuse out of hand.

The next question was suggested by a disagreement over whether or not to deceive a failing patient about the death of a loved one: "What's happiness, anyway?" Grisez's answer is that our real happiness is not a matter of contentment or even euphoria. Nor is happiness episodic. Rather, we are happy to the extent that we participate in the basic goods, the constituents of our flourishing. We are happy to the degree that the choices fashioning our characters are rightly ordered to these goods. Because knowledge is a basic good, any attack on our knowing the truth is morally wrong. Intentionally deceiving another is wrong. Such deception undercuts happiness far more radically than does learning even very bad news. The person deceived is denied the truth. The deceiver undercuts his or her own authenticity — and the community between the two people is impeded.

The third question was triggered by a judge's puzzlement over "cultural breaks" between the larger society and believers in faith healing: "Are there universal moral truths?" Grisez's answer is in the affirmative. Each person is made in God's image. Thus at the most fundamental level, we share a dynamic human nature that fulfills its potential by realizing a range of identifiable basic goods. Indeed, it is these goods upon which universal human rights are grounded. Of course, different cultures develop different strategies for promoting the goods, and these strategies should be respected. Nonetheless, there are also cultural defects that a wider experience of human nature reveals. Slavery is one example, sexism another. In the case that prompted the judge's query, Grisez would argue that each person has a right to basic health care and that even a parent's religious convictions cannot override this.

The fourth question, occasioned by a visit to a cancer hospice, was "Are there moral absolutes?" An anguished plea for euthanasia might prompt such a query about even the cherished medical dictum *primum non nocere*, "first of all, do no harm." Grisez would say that there are moral absolutes for the same reason that there are inalienable rights. Each corresponds to a basic good that cannot be attacked either by another or by oneself without assailing a fundamental dimension of one's person. Since life is just such a basic good, even voluntary euthanasia violates the person. For the same reason, self-mutilation is a violation, as is reckless risking of injury. By contrast, a legitimate organ donation — constructive in its very character — leaves the donor's basic physical integrity intact. What is at stake here is a right to life grounded in the very dignity of the person.

Our fifth question was prompted by the offer of an obstetrical post requiring one to do abortions. The question asks: "When does life begin?" It immediately suggests another: "When does life end?" In our culture both questions are posed with increasing urgency. But, strictly speaking, neither begins as an ethical question. Instead, each is at once scientific and metaphysical. When the metaphysical side predominates, the question is really, "Is this a *person* yet — or still?" For Grisez, to be a person is to be a *kind* of being, the kind that either is or has the potential to be a rational agent. Any "living, human individual" meets this criterion (1970a: 416). With special reference to a person's coming to be, Grisez argues that "if a human activated ovum has in itself the epigenetic primordia of a human body normal enough to be the organic basis of at least some intellectual act, that activated ovum is a person" (1989a: 21). By "epigenetic primordia" Grisez means the most rudimentary forms from which a body or, more specifically, an organ — for example, the brain — develops.

In particular cases of doubt about personhood, we ought to err on the side of caution when once we turn from metaphysical speculation to ethical analysis. Thus Grisez maintains, "To be willing to kill what for all one knows is a person is to be willing to kill a person. Hence, in making moral judgments the unborn should be considered persons from the beginning — their lives instances of innocent human life" (1989a: 23). Thus any living human being ought to be counted as a person. (A Christian who looks to the resurrection anticipates a future in which even the most defective human beings will realize a fully human and personal potential.) Consider two cases in particular: a brain-damaged person and an anencephalic baby. In the first case the individual remains a person, though defective. Personhood, after all, is not a stage but a kind. And Grisez argues, since an anencephalic baby once had the requisite epigenetic primordia (subsequently compromised *in utero*), it shares the same status as a newly brain-damaged person.

The sixth of our probing questions was "What proportion of our resources can we direct to health care?" The beleaguered hospital director who asked it was immediately challenged by the counterquestion "How much is a human life worth?" Grisez would argue that his answer to the latter helps structure his reply to the former. Because human life is priceless, we share a right to life. A right to ordinary health care flows from this right. Still a society's resources might be sharply limited. In the United States, ordinary health care involves a right to kidney dialysis. In India it does not. Nor need this difference imply some moral disorder on India's part. It might simply illustrate that even at the social level it is not always possible to pursue all of the basic goods equally. What obligations affluent countries have to less developed nations is a related question. Any society that has more resources than it needs to realize the basic goods has a *prima facie* obligation to help meet the pressing needs of less developed countries. In scriptural language, we are our brother's keeper.

169

Finally, we come to the seventh and last of our questions. Suppose that an organization of medical professionals finds that a majority of its members thinks abortion morally wrong. Should the organization file an *amicus curiae* brief arguing for overturning *Roe v. Wade* when next the Supreme Court addresses the abortion question? Or suppose that this organization comes to a majority decision that euthanasia is immoral. Should it work for legal restrictions on abortion or the prohibition of euthanasia? Or, as some would surely insist, should public policy make "personal choice" paramount?

Grisez would address such questions by drawing on a pair of guiding considerations. Common sense and long experience tell us that though some actions can be wrong, legally prohibiting them only makes matters worse. Thus Aquinas wisely taught that civil law properly "does not lay upon the multitude of imperfect people the burdens of those who are already virtuous, namely, that they should abstain from all evil" (*Summa Theologiae*, II-I, q.96, a.2). This country's dismal experience with Prohibition offers a handy example.

But another principle is equally important, though it must be prefaced with an account of the political order's functioning. The state seeks the common good; not to do so would forfeit its very legitimacy. But the common good is not simply the utilitarian's maximization of pleasure over pain, since maximizing pleasure might well entail the mistreatment of a minority. The common good must include the good of all. No one, and surely no innocent person, is expendable. As a result, the state rightfully uses legal sanctions to realize and protect this good. Our second principle is that the law must protect the basic goods of all.

Grisez would argue that the law ought always to reject the intentional taking of innocent human life. (Indeed, he would go further. We ought never intentionally to take human life. This rules out capital punishment — but not self-defense, in which one intends to "stop" but not to kill the aggressor [1983: 220; 1970b: 66-72].) Therefore, the law ought to prohibit both euthanasia and abortion. Respecting the fundamental right to life is our common obligation, not just the special duty of the few. Just what form legal sanctions would take is another matter. For a start, sanctions seem more properly directed at those who profit from the taking of life rather than at those whose circumstances seem almost to impel them to a lethal solution to their predicaments.

Earlier I suggested that we have all become familiar with the set of "questions overheard" that might well serve as a practical introduction to, and test of, Germain Grisez's challenging version of natural law ethics. Taken together, our probing questions do give a sense of the larger shape of his systematic moral perspective. Before turning to some significant objections to Grisez's approach, I would like to consider a particular bioethical problem that is rightly receiving an increasing amount of attention and sketch Grisez's evolving analysis of this problem.

A Test Case: Feeding and Hydrating

Many ethicists would agree that the quality of a patient's life would have a great bearing on whether or not feeding and hydrating ought to be continued, especially if feeding tubes are required. After all, they reason, life is a good. But it is not an intrinsic, much less an absolute, good. Of far more value is the patient's personhood or, alternatively, his or her relational capacity. But suppose our patient is in a persistent vegetative state, or severely retarded, or the victim of some mentally incapacitating disorder such as Alzheimer's. Then we have, at most, the remnants of a person. Moreover, though to cut off feeding and hydrating would result in death, to rely on tubes is to resort to extraordinary means. It is never necessary to employ such means. Indeed, in a context of scarce medical resources, it may be socially irresponsible to do so.

For this last reason, Germain Grisez was at one time inclined to suppose that providing nutrition and hydration in such cases would not be necessary. Thus he held that "if a patient is not in imminent danger of death but is in an irreversible coma . . . life support care more sophisticated than ordinary nursing care . . . exceeds a permanently comatose person's fair share of available facilities and services" (1986: 49). More recently, however, Grisez has come to the opposite conclusion, in part because he now considers tubal feeding and hydration neither complicated nor expensive. In a recent document coordinated by William E. May, Grisez supported the view that there is a strong presumption in favor of such treatment. The document reached the conclusion that "in the ordinary circumstances of life in our society today, it is not morally right, nor ought it to be legally permissible, to withhold or withdraw nutrition and hydration provided by artificial means to the permanently unconscious or other categories of seriously debilitated but nonterminal persons. Rather, food and fluids are universally needed

171

for the preservation of life, and can generally be provided without the burdens and expense of more aggressive means of supporting life" (1987: 211).

In dismissing quality-of-life considerations, Grisez is consistent with his own long-standing rejection of a supposed dualism between the human being and the human person. We are not, he insists, two things — a human being *and* a person — somehow temporarily conjoined. For Grisez, as we have seen, to be a person is to be a kind of being, not simply to have a certain function or to be at a certain stage. Human life is always personal, although it may not always manifest the distinctively personal traits of reason and communication. Again, a person's life is an intrinsic good. Instrumental goods are distinct from the unity of the person. But one's very life is not distinct from the person one is — a point that Grisez has made in other contexts where killing is at issue (1987a: 309). The general moral implication of this argument is clear: to neglect a person's life is to neglect the person.

In applying this finding to the issue of feeding and hydrating, we must carefully distinguish between the burden of care and the burden of life. The life of a person in a persistent vegetative state is a burden. It is, to be sure, often more of a burden for the caretakers than for the patient. But the burden of care is another matter altogether. In ordinary cases tubal feeding and nutrition maintain the patient's life, which remains a good in itself, without placing some new burden of treatment on the patient. Nor is this form of care excessively costly or invasive.

Failing to provide an ordinary means of care is to dissolve the distinction between not treating and killing. When we do not provide ordinary treatment, our intention comes perilously close to — if not identical with — that of the person who simply kills a patient. When this happens, Grisez would argue, we have become deaf to the plea of the Second Vatican Council: "Feed the man dying of hunger, because if you do not feed him you have killed him" (Pastoral Constitution on the Church in the Modern World, n. 69).

Admittedly, there are exceptions. It may be that the very providing of nutrition and hydration becomes painful or seriously invasive. In the stages just prior to death, a person may not be able to absorb the food and liquid we provide. In such cases the treatment becomes pointless because it offers the patient no benefit. But ordinarily we are obliged to feed and hydrate those who cannot care for themselves. Life itself is a personal good, not a kind of neutral "stepping stone" to a higher plane where, for the first time, ethical values come into play. Because Grisez sees human life as necessarily personal, he refuses to depersonalize the permanently unconscious. Only by doing so can our society rationalize killing them, by commission or omission.

Grisez's recent and full account of how he has come to his new position on feeding and hydration has raised a fresh point of dispute. In his newest analysis, he makes clear that in addition to the obvious cases where feeding and hydration are not required — where they would not sustain life, where they would add to the patient's burden, where a society's resources would be unfairly drained by them — there is a fourth exempting case. "Competent persons who envisage the situation of being comatose, and who clearly and freely reject food in that situation should it ever come about, need not be choosing to kill themselves. They can, instead, be choosing both to avoid being kept alive by a method toward which they feel psychological repugnance and to free others of the cost of caring for them" (1989b: 176). If such informed prior consent has been adequately communicated, we can justifiably eschew artificial feeding and hydration. In respecting such a request, we affirm the dignity of the person who made it.

At least two problems arise with this further nuancing of Grisez's view. The first is that it seems unfairly to penalize those who through no fault of their own fail to communicate their consent. The second is whether or not such a consent is reasonable, since it effectively forfeits the personal good of one's own life.

To the first objection one might reply that in the present cultural context, where the sanctity of life is increasingly precarious, Grisez is probably right to insist on a fully communicated consent. I am not at all sure, however, that he can meet the second objection, since in his view one is not justified in rejecting the ordinary means of preserving life. It is, in addition, not clear how one's prior psychological repugnance to a means of care that at the time of its use might not be repugnant can be a decisive factor. Nor is it clear why the psychological repugnance of one's caretakers should be decisive. Moreover, what we take to be psychologically repugnant ought to be acknowledged but not simply accepted uncritically. For in a culture in which any dependence on others is often wrongly seen as a forfeiture of human dignity, it may well be that we have become conditioned to feel as demeaning what in fact is not. The truth is, of course, that human beings in countless ways all depend on one another.

However Grisez might respond to this particular pair of objections, his analysis of the issue will doubtless contribute to, and in turn be affected by, our heightened moral and legal concern over artificial feeding and hydration. His contributions, we can safely predict, will be provocative. In particular, the second volume of his major work, *The Way of the Lord Jesus,* is now nearing publication, and it promises to focus on a wide range of critical moral questions. While many will appreciate Grisez's forthrightness, others will hesitate to accept such definite answers. Ours is an intellectual milieu that often seems to prefer questions without answers — and so without confrontations either.

Criticism and Response

Among the broader criticisms that Germain Grisez's natural law ethics encounters, the most frequent objection is the consequentialist or pro-portionalist charge that being sensitive to the results of our acts occasionally must lead us to act against a basic good. Sometimes, then, whether in medicine or war, we are justified in intentionally ending an innocent life.

Grisez's response to this is both philosophical and theological. First, he challenges the consequentialists to give us some objective means of ranking the basic goods or even particular instances of a basic good. Historically the temptation to kill the one, or the few, to save the many has been constant. Scripture offers a chilling precedent in the Sanhedrin's Caiaphas, who asks, "Can you not see that it is better to have one man die than to have the whole nation destroyed?" (John 11:50). Only in modernity has this temptation cloaked itself with ethical respectability. Second, from the perspective of faith we see that it can never be justifiable intentionally to attack a basic good, since to do so is to attack the person — who is made in God's image.

Another common objection is that a Christian natural law perspective like Grisez's must recognize that our culture is characterized by ethical pluralism — a pluralism that has found room for utilitarians as well as natural law thinkers, for ethical subjectivists as well as those who argue for universal moral norms, for moral skeptics as well as those who claim to have found the contours of important moral truths. More to the point, this line of criticism continues, our society cannot function unless this ethical pluralism is given its head. Political democracy depends on moral heterogeneity. Perhaps some religious traditions can require more. American society, however, must be content with a moral minimum. Ethics must be pragmatically restrained.

Grisez's short answer is that ethical reflection aims for moral truth, not political equilibrium. But there is a second and equally important reply. It is not at all obvious that democratic society can sustain itself on a kind of ethical lowest common denominator. The political order can scarcely claim to pursue the common good if there is no shared vision of that good. Where democracy already is precarious, is it not largely because there is no shared appreciation of what is valuable for human nature? Cultures where democracy fails are those that cannot recognize people's intrinsic worth. Grisez's natural law system is not a threat to pluralism. Rather, it offers a promising articulation of a moral order that makes possible democratic politics.

A final objection is harder to state, though perhaps widely felt. Roughly it is the following: "In the end moral theory is artificial and inadequate, especially when it tries to be logical and systematic. After all, we live not by abstract principles but by the wisdom of religious traditions or by the light of morally sensitive consciences. Virtuous people don't need moral theory, and vicious people ignore it."

In a less perplexed time, Grisez would have a certain sympathy for such impatience. Natural law ethics begins, after all, by reflecting on the sense of human good that one finds in the great religions and in the sensitive consciences of decent people. But our times are hugely perplexing. In such periods the great religious traditions encourage reflection on their teachings; they survive by growing in the light of such reflection. In such times, too, the sensitive conscience expresses itself in the analysis and application of carefully articulated moral principles. Indeed, a measure of the virtuous person is a commitment to careful reflection on just what the virtues require of us. Hence, natural law ethics is not a creature of academic speculation. Rather, it grows out of sustained examination of the demands of the moral life.

A Second Opinion

In retrospect, this century will impress its students as a time of deep and protracted crises. In such a time, ethical analysis, in the larger context of Christian faith, will generate its own contribution of tension and ambiguity. But human nature has not become an unfathomable mystery. The pilgrimage of faith has the same end now as it has always had: a coming to share in God's own life.

While we are on this pilgrimage, our moral imperative is full obedience to God's will, a will that is at once legislative and creative. As a moral theologian, Grisez pays special attention to God's legislative will. As a moral philosopher, he attends to the human nature that is a splendid though flawed part of God's creation — a testimony to God's creative will. Because Grisez is both theologian and philosopher, his work combines a depth of vision and a logical rigor that are too rarely brought together. At the same time, his dual role will cause some to consider his vision ungrounded and others to find his logical rigor restrictive.

Such judgments are regrettable if they lead to a facile and convenient dismissal. But the loss will be the critics' own. Our era has already seen too much intellectual compartmentalization. Has it not also witnessed, partly as a consequence, a widespread failure of moral and intellectual nerve? A close study of Germain Grisez's natural law ethics might afford us just the second opinion we need to improve our chances for working through the daunting bioethical quandaries we so routinely face.

References

Aquinas, Thomas. 1945. *Summa Theologiae.* Benzinger Brothers.

Grisez, Germain. 1964. *Contraception and the Natural Law.* Milwaukee: Bruce Publishing.

———. 1970a. *Abortion: The Myths, the Realities, and the Arguments.* New York: Corpus Books.

———. 1970b. "Toward a Consistent Natural Law Ethics of Killing." *American Journal of Jurisprudence* 15: 64-96.

———. 1979. *Life and Death with Liberty and Justice,* with Joseph M. Boyle, Jr. Notre Dame and London: University of Notre Dame Press.

———. 1983. *The Way of the Lord Jesus,* vol. 1 of *Christian Moral Principles,* with the help of Joseph M. Boyle, Jr., Basil Cole, O.P., John M. Finnis, John A. Geinzer, Jeanette Grisez, Robert G. Kennedy, Patrick Lee, William E. May, and Russell Shaw. Chicago: Franciscan Herald Press.

———. 1986. "A Christian Ethics of Limiting Medical Treatment: Guidelines for Patients, Proxy Decision Makers and Counselors." In *Pope John Paul II Lecture Series in Bioethics,* 35-56. New Britain, Conn.: Mariel Publications.

————. 1989a. "Should Nutrition and Hydration Be Provided to Permanently Unconscious and Other Mentally Disabled Persons?" *Issues in Law and Medicine* 5, no. 2 (Fall): 165-79.

————. 1989b. "When Do People Begin?" In *Proceedings of the American Catholic Philosophical Association.*

Grisez, Germain, John M. Finnis, and Joseph M. Boyle, Jr. 1987a. *Nuclear Deterrence, Morality and Realism.* Oxford and New York: Oxford University Press.

Grisez, Germain, Joseph M. Boyle, Jr., and John M. Finnis. 1987b. "Practical Principles, Moral Truth, and Ultimate Ends." *American Journal of Jurisprudence* 32: 99-151.

Hanink, James, and Gary Mar. 1987. "What Euthyphro Couldn't Have Said." *Faith and Philosophy* 4, no. 3 (July): 241-61.

May, William E. (Coordinator, Drafting Committee). 1987. "Feeding and Hydrating the Permanently Unconscious and Other Vulnerable Persons." *Issues in Law and Medicine* 3, no. 3 (Winter): 203-17.

Ramsey, Paul. 1978. *Ethics at the Edges of Life.* New Haven: Yale University Press.

ON IMMANUEL JAKOBOVITS

Bringing the Ancient Word to the Modern World

MARC A. GELLMAN

I. Biographical Sketch

AT THIS time of his impending retirement from the office of the Chief Rabbinate of Great Britain and the Commonwealth, at the occasion of his being awarded the Templeton Prize, and in tribute to the unique scope and vigor of his life and work, it is fitting and proper to recognize and acknowledge the contribution of Rabbi Immanuel Jakobovits, a remarkable Jewish leader, Jewish thinker, and Jewish teacher who was clearly responsible for opening up the discipline of Jewish medical ethics.

Rabbi Immanuel Jakobovits ("Lord Jakobovits," his official title following his elevation to the peerage in 1988, remains, for me at least, just a touch heretical for an essay with theological overtones!) opened the field of Jewish medical ethics first with his doctoral dissertation for Jews' College in London in 1955 and later with the publication of its expanded version in 1959 under the title *Jewish Medical Ethics*. This work not only was the first to use the term *Jewish medical ethics* but also was the first to collect and analyze the full range of classic Jewish legal sources on some of the emerging issues of medical ethics. In 1975 a fourth edition of the book was published with a new chapter, "Recent Developments in Jewish Medical Ethics," which surveyed the explosion of interest in medical ethics since 1959.

Although this book remains his only one on medical ethics, his

178

many essays, speeches, and reviews elaborate and expand on that earlier work. Rabbi Jakobovits has also done much to help encourage particularly Israeli scholars to contribute to this field. In his honor, a chair in Jewish medical ethics has been established at the Ben Gurion University of the Negev.

One must, first off, admire Rabbi Jakobovits's prescience. When he began his work in the 1950s, the emergence of medical ethics as an important interdisciplinary field of interest to philosophers, lawyers, physicians, and theologians was fully a decade away.[1] No doubt his own wide range of interests and obligations, from the pastoral responsibilities of a pulpit rabbi to the intellectual challenge of defending the contemporary relevance of Orthodox Judaism, all predisposed him to this new area of contact and conflict between an inherited ancient faith and the ethical problems of modern medical science.

His concern for the central issues facing modern people, and thus modern Jews, was not limited to his ground-breaking work in medical ethics. His collected essays, *The Timely and the Timeless: Jews, Judaism and Society in a Storm-tossed Decade* (1989), and also his *Journal of a Rabbi* (1966) reveal an intellect of extraordinary scope and courage. Topics dealt with by Rabbi Jakobovits are as diverse, controversial, and difficult as war and peace with the Palestinians, the religious significance of the state of Israel, intermarriage, the strengths and weaknesses of Jewish orthodoxy, and (that thorny and much debated problem) the applicability of Jewish ritual laws for space travelers.

Through essays in Jewish journals and through his annual Passover and New Year's broadcasts in Great Britain, Rabbi Jakobovits was a tireless and often controversial contributor to the debates in the Jewish world on Israeli political life, the religious practices of the state of Israel, and the state of world Jewry. Rabbi Jakobovits persevered in his efforts to bring Jewish values to bear on the problems of the modern world.

This mix of practical and theoretical interests reflected Rabbi Jakobovits's professional life. Eschewing the life of a cloistered scholar,

---

1. I believe that the ground swell of social notice of this new source of ethical dilemmas began with the revolutionary 1967 report of the ad hoc committee of the Harvard Medical School on new criteria for brain death. The development of clinically reliable transplant procedures, the concern for the rights of subjects in medical experimentation, and the reversal of the existing abortion laws in *Roe v. Wade* and *Doe v. Bolton* were in succession the next causal factors for the rise of interest in the field of medical ethics, factors that coalesced between 1967 and 1978.

he became an active pulpit rabbi. Ordained at age 20 after fleeing Hitler's Germany and his hometown of Konigsberg, Rabbi Jakobovits first served congregations in London from 1941 to 1949 (Abramson 1989: 377). In 1949 he became Chief Rabbi of Ireland, where he served until 1958. He lived in America from 1958 to 1967 following his election to the pulpit of the prestigious Fifth Avenue Synagogue in Manhattan.

During this time in New York, Rabbi Jakobovits helped create one of the most important and unique medical ethics groups in the world, the Medical Ethics Committee of the Federation of Jewish Philanthropies of Greater New York. The committee of the United Jewish Appeal (UJA) Federation of New York was the first and still remains one of the few Jewish medical ethics committees in the world to seek representation from all branches of Judaism and from the legal and medical professions.

In 1963 and 1965 he coauthored the first two editions of *A Hospital Compendium: A Guide to Jewish Moral and Religious Principles in Hospital Practice.* This work, compiled by Rabbi Jakobovits and the committee of physicians and rabbis, was first conceived of as merely a practical resource for hospital professionals to help them deal with some of the ritual and, to a lesser extent, the medical ethical problems arising in the care of Orthodox Jewish patients. The committee quickly moved beyond the relatively modest aims of its first publication and soon produced, under the editorship of Rabbi Moshe Tendler of Yeshiva University, the driving intellectual force of the committee after the departure of Rabbi Jakobovits for England, a *Compendium of Jewish Medical Ethics,* which addressed many controversial and contemporary issues. More than 100,000 copies of the *Compendium* (now in its sixth edition) are in print.[2] As the present chairman of that committee, I can see firsthand the results that Rabbi Jakobovits's work and planning still produce. I regret his departure for England and his appointment as Chief Rabbi of Great Britain and the Commonwealth in 1967. His responsibilities

2. The compendium is now called the *Compendium on Medical Ethics* and has continued to evolve. As the present chairman of the medical ethics committee, I am constantly impressed by the vision of Rabbi Jakobovits in bringing together rabbis, physicians, attorneys, and philosophers from all branches of Judaism to discuss and debate topics of Jewish medical ethics. The committee is a unique and productive example of the results of teamwork in doing work in this field. The *Compendium* can be obtained by writing the Federation of Jewish Philanthropies, 130 East 59th Street, New York, N.Y. 10022.

have surely limited the time he could devote to scholarly writing in the field he clearly prepared.

In this essay I will examine Jakobovits's conception of the project of Jewish medical ethics. This field, a unique intellectual and theological hybrid, tests the flexibility and vitality of Jewish law in addressing new and complex moral issues in medical science as well as the intellectual credibility of Jewish moral reasoning in the realm of modern normative ethical thinking.

Even though it is not true, there are good reasons to suppose at the outset that Judaism would have little to say about the problems of modern medical ethics. After all, a tradition that emerged just as humankind was mastering the art of smelting iron could hardly be blamed for not having a coherent view of heart transplantation, in vitro fertilization, or genetic engineering. Even an issue such as abortion, which was dealt with in Jewish legal tradition, was considered when there was no knowledge of genetics and only a minimal ability to save a mother or a child from any medical complication.

Jakobovits, and every Jewish thinker who has ever wished to contribute meaningfully to the field of medical ethics, first had to establish that this ancient legal and spiritual tradition called Judaism had a tradition of legal and narrative teachings about medical ethical issues. Not only was it imperative that those teachings be collected and systematized, but also the values and legal hermeneutics of that tradition had to be carefully delineated so that rulings covering new and unforeseen medical ethical issues could be made.

Collecting Jewish legal texts and then explicating them in philosophically accessible language is a tall order. To do medical ethics properly one must be well grounded in law, medicine, and philosophy. To that, add the requirement that one be conversant with the entire warp and woof of Jewish law and commentaries, and it becomes immediately evident that this is a field no single person could conceivably master even in a few lifetimes. For this reason, some have entered the field with primary training as physicians and with a secondary knowledge of Jewish law.[3] Still others, sensitive to the philosophical demands of this

3. Dr. Fred Rosner, director of medicine at Queens Hospital Center and professor of medicine at the State University of New York, is a good example of this approach. His important contributions to the field of Jewish medical ethics include *Modern Medicine and Jewish Law* and *Modern Medicine and Jewish Ethics,* as well as *Jewish Bioethics,* with Rabbi J. David Bleich.

work, have entered the field of Jewish medical ethics as professionally trained philosophers with a personal exposure to Jewish law and an acquired specialty in medical ethics.[4] However, by far the largest group of people doing Jewish medical ethics today are rabbis, experts in Jewish law who must augment laypersons' knowledge of medicine with non-philosophers' knowledge of moral philosophy.[5] It is in no small measure due to the work of Jakobovits that rabbis and not Jewish physicians or Jewish philosophers have defined the field as it exists today.

If what follows seems at points to imply Rabbi Jakobovits was not completely successful in his project, it is meant as no disparagement. Jakobovits can hardly be faulted for not being an *homo universalis*. He

4. Baruch Brody, the Leon Jaworski Professor of Biomedical Ethics and the director of the Center for Ethics, Medicine and Public Issues at Baylor College of Medicine, is by far the most able contemporary philosopher to consider Jewish issues in his work. Brody's unique skills make him the most philosophically literate practitioner of Jewish medical ethics today. Though not a rabbi, his knowledge of the Jewish legal literature is very deep. In his early work *Abortion and the Sanctity of Human Life: A Philosophical View,* he uses sources in the Jewish legal literature to augment his general arguments. Recently, as he has moved exclusively into medical ethics, he has taken up the challenge of offering a philosophical critique of modern Orthodox rabbis and their approach to Jewish medical ethics. See, for example, his excellent essay "A Historical Introduction to Jewish Casuistry on Suicide and Euthanasia" (1989). And for more general issues relating to the process of doing Jewish medical ethics see his 1983 essay, "The Use of Halakhic Material in Discussions of Medical Ethics," and his recent book, *Life and Death Decision-Making.*

5. The two dominant figures among the Orthodox rabbinate in the field of medical ethics today are Rabbi J. David Bleich and Rabbi Moshe Tendler, both of Yeshiva University in New York. Bleich has training in law, Tendler in biology. Bleich is the author of three volumes of *Contemporary Halakhic Problems* and *Judaism and Healing.* He is the coeditor with Dr. Fred Rosner of *Jewish Bioethics.* Moshe Tendler was responsible for editing and authoring substantial segments of the fifth edition of the *Compendium of Medical Ethics,* published by the UJA-Federation of New York. He has published a number of scholarly articles in the field (see, e.g., Tendler 1968). These men have continued to expand the field of Jewish medical ethics along the lines Rabbi Jakobovits established. A valuable journal, accessible to the English reader, that presents new opinions of Orthodox Jewish scholars and rabbis regarding a variety of Jewish legal and ethical questions is *Proceedings of the Association of Orthodox Jewish Scientists* (Sepher-Hermon Press, New York). Conservative rabbis have also contributed to the field, notable among them David Novak, Seymour Siegel, Isaac Klein, and especially David Feldman, whose book *Birth Control in Jewish Law* remains a classic work on Jewish views of marital relations, contraception, and abortion. Rabbi Seymour Siegel and Rabbi David Gordis have also written in this field. Among Reform rabbis who have contributed are Solomon Freehof, who has addressed a variety of bioethical issues in his collected works of Reform responsa, and continuing the work of Rabbi Freehof, Walter Jacob. Also see Rabbi Arnold Wolf's excellent essay "Judaism on Medicine" (1976).

brings to this task more than enough tools to solidify his position as one of the most important Jewish scholars and interpreters of our time. The demands of Jewish medical ethics are extraordinary, and the dialogue between religion and philosophy on any topic is always in search of common ground and always frustrated in large or small measure in that search (Fackenheim 1973). One can say without a doubt that Immanuel Jakobovits was the first really to begin to systematically address the varied and challenging elements of Jewish medical ethics in a way intended for both scholar and layperson, for both Jew and Gentile. Every Jewish scholar of medical ethics will be eternally in his debt for his pioneering work.

Rabbi Jakobovits is part of an ancient, if sparsely populated, tradition of Jewish thinkers who intend as their audience not just the believing Jewish community but the broader secular world as well. One of his intellectual and spiritual predecessors was the great medieval Jewish philosopher Moses Maimonides. Perhaps Maimonides was the last human being fully qualified in law, medicine, philosophy, theology, and Jewish law for the project of Jewish medical ethics. The modern explosion of knowledge has made such comprehensive intellectual mastery impossible. Maimonides attempted for the Jewish community the great synthesis of reason and revelation, of Greek and Jewish thought, in his philosophical work, *The Guide for the Perplexed,* and developed Jewish legal theory in his code of Jewish law, the *Mishna Torah.*[6]

Another important spiritual and intellectual mentor for Jakobovits was the towering figure of German Jewish orthodoxy before World War I, Rabbi Samson Raphael Hirsch. Rabbi Hirsch, a literate, learned, and cultured German Jew, engaged in polemics with the leadership of the new Reform movement in Judaism, bringing to the debate a vision of an Orthodox Judaism that could defend itself in modern terms without assimilating into that world. Hirsch held to a Judaism that could transmit in modern language and idiom the truths of the ancient faith and laws without apology and without surrender of the tradition. Rabbi Jakobovits saw in Hirsch a model of the modern Orthodox Jew.[7]

---

6. See his comparison of Rabbi Yosef Karo and Maimonides (Jakobovits 1989: 314-17) for a clear example of the way Jakobovits lauds and favors Maimonides's rational approach to Jewish law.

7. His admiration for Hirsch is seen clearly in a lecture delivered at Jews' College, London, 16 June 1971, and included in the collection *The Timely and the Timeless.*

Maimonides and Hirsch gave Jakobovits his starting point for his project: *Any authentic Jewish contribution to medical ethics and indeed to modern thought must begin from and must be rooted in the tradition of Jewish law.* For Jakobovits, law, *halacha,* and not story, *aggada,* is the central defining element of Judaism, and thus the Jewish contribution to medical ethics must begin from its legal sources. In the Judaism Jakobovits knows, abstract ideas are instantiated in law, general beliefs find particular form in law, and the Jewish community as a whole was and, according to Jakobovits, ought to remain a community formed by laws. As such it is the authority of the Jewish jurist, the *posek,* that is critical, not the cogency of moral reasoning based on some abstracted principles. Jewish moral thinking, according to Jakobovits, leads to the *posek* and not to the philosopher. In an interview he commented on those who try to engage moral problems from an abstract perspective:

> When I read letters, say, of Jewish participation in debates on moral problems such as abortion or euthanasia, which happen to be areas of special interest to me, I find that those who participate on the universalist basis, on the general basis, have no Jewish insights or commitments to offer whatsoever. In fact, they are usually ignorant of the Jewish stand in these areas. (Fein 1987: 320)

Jewish law has, Jakobovits is quick to acknowledge, universalist elements, but the method and the consequence of Jewish moral reasoning flow from the laws through the ancient process of authorized Orthodox interpretation of the laws to new laws for new circumstances, and not, as some liberal Jewish thinkers would have it, from the laws to their universal substrate and from there to new laws.

Therefore, the first task he set himself was to survey all relevant Jewish laws pertaining to medical ethics, and then, through a close legal exegesis, to derive new laws for new circumstances. This form of moral reasoning is not easily accessible nor is it clearly a form of moral reasoning for those with predilections for philosophical autonomy, but it is the way Jews have decided between right and wrong for 2,000 years. Rabbi Jakobovits is ready to move the focus of Jewish law into the new realm of medical ethics, but he is not willing to alter the Jewish legal process, which has confronted novelty before without surrendering the ancient way.

II. Accommodating Change

Any theologically based legal system like Orthodox Judaism faces the central methodological problem of explaining changes in the law over time. The revelation to Moses on Mt. Sinai was once believed to be perfect and free of contradictions, valid for all time. However, changes in historical circumstance refuted that belief. In the rabbinic period, the concept of an oral law — believed to have been revealed to Moses along with the written law on Mt. Sinai — provided the theological flexibility that permitted Judaism to accommodate changes in the law and in belief. By giving the Hebrew Bible and the Talmud relatively equal theological status, the authenticity of rabbinic theological and legal innovations was vouchsafed.

The same theological move, however, could not be made over and over throughout Jewish history. From the sixth to the twelfth centuries only one basic reformulation of the Jewish legal corpus occurred; after this code, the *shulhan aruch,* no universally binding code of Jewish law was ever accepted. A new form of Jewish legal creativity arose, the responsa. These were questions submitted to individual rabbis and answers sent back to the individual petitioner. The responsa literature, particularly of the postwar period, is the richest source of Jewish laws on medical ethics.

These responsa do not have the legal authority of the Talmud or Bible or codes, but they served (as they still do) as the mechanism for innovation and accommodation in Orthodox Judaism during a period when Jewish legal creativity was needed but no Orthodox rabbi had sufficient authority to rule for the whole Jewish world. Responsa serve a theological need, because in a private letter not intending to establish universal Jewish legal norms, a rabbi is freer to innovate than he would be in a full and public reformulation of Jewish law. Furthermore, these responsa usually conclude with the theologically useful caveat, "the matter needs more investigation." In this way the *posek,* the rabbinic jurist, is further protected against the charge of altering the previous legal sources and is also not forced to reconcile his responsum with those of other rabbis who might have ruled in a contrary fashion.

Medical questions in Jewish law present a very special problem. Ancient Jewish laws about holiday observance, ritual practice, or rites of passage are never really confronted by the necessity for change. However, the Bible and the Talmud are not just works of theology or of ritual

185

or of life cycle events. They also reflect the scientific knowledge of their time, and that knowledge was obviously primitive. To continue to observe holidays that reflect the ancient agricultural cycle in the land of Israel may seem irrelevant to some, but it is hardly dangerous. But many of the medical laws of the Bible and the Talmud are simply wrong and injurious to health if followed. In the Jewish laws concerning healing, change was imperative.

Jakobovits addresses the problem of change at the outset of his study. He points to certain tendencies in the Jewish legal tradition itself to justify changes in Jewish medical laws. He finds in the tradition medieval rabbis who taught that changes in nature brought about by God justify corresponding changes in the law, which reflects nature (Jakobovits 1975: xxxviii). By this logic it is not the revelation but rather God through nature who changes, and this removes the thorny theological problem of change in a revealed corpus of law.

In addition to the "changes in nature" principle that facilitated changes in the law, Jakobovits finds in the tradition the additional legal principle of "we are no longer competent experts" (1975: xli). This legal hermeneutic enabled rabbis to ignore medically outdated rulings of the Bible and Talmud by stating that the expertise to do the tests required in these ancient texts was no longer possessed by Jews of their time, and therefore there was justification for following the dictates of modern medicine in accepted clinical procedures.

The resolution of the problem of change was forced on Orthodox Judaism by medical science more than by any other challenge. Orthodox teachings on Jewish rituals can resist changes quite successfully because rituals do not generally present life and death choices, but not so Jewish laws concerning illness and healing. In this arena, the advances in medical science had to be acknowledged. The powerful Jewish value of the sanctity of human life as well as the ancient principle that most laws can be violated to save a life provide a basis for changing Jewish law to promote healing and save lives. In general that has been precisely the approach of Orthodox rabbinic teachings toward medical science, and it is at the heart of Jakobovits's modern Orthodox project as well. He simply does not believe or concede that the practice of medicine conflicts with Jewish teachings in any fundamental way. He believes that "Jewish medical ethics, though commanding no literature of its own, is a subject of broad dimensions, built on an abundance of literary material, that the sources we shall utilize do not necessarily reflect the outlook of the time of their composition, and that the medico-religious views recorded in them are, in certain respects, flexible enough to allow for continuous revision and adjustment" (1975: xlii). In fact, Judaism is nearly univocal in its endorsement of the healing arts (Jakobovits 1975: 303 n. 5).[8]

This liberal view may strike some as inconsistent with the biblical belief that God punishes sins in this life and that illness and suffering are forms of this divine punishment. These two beliefs seem to lead to the conclusion that medical healing is a religiously unjustified thwarting of God's providence. Thus, Jakobovits also had to overcome the theological obstacle of explaining to physicians and skeptical theologians why Judaism had no religious problem endorsing medical healing as a commandment from God.

Judaism, Jakobovits indicates, focuses on the preciousness of life, the sanctity of life, and therefore anything that preserves life is in conformity with the essential and foundational teachings of Judaism. The Talmud speaks the eloquent and pervasive Jewish truth, "He who saves one life is as if he had saved an entire world."

In philosophical terms, the Jewish tradition endorses the ancient beliefs that God punishes sins in this life and that illness and suffering are forms of that punishment, while still rejecting the conclusion that medical healing is religiously unjustified. The tradition seems to be claiming that one can accept illness as punishment but accept the overriding belief in the sanctity of life as permitting the alleviation of suffering and illness to the extent possible.

These methodological problems having been resolved, the next ten chapters of *Jewish Medical Ethics* cover the general attitude of Judaism toward healing. Superstitious cures, danger to life, the sick and their treatment — all are discussed, but no pressing contemporary ethical issues emerge in fully the first half of the book. Jakobovits seems content to survey the Jewish approach to medicine in general, rather than the Jewish approach to specific medical ethical issues. Even when he turns in chapter 11 to such an important area of moral conflict as the care of dying patients, ethical issues are given short shrift.

For a book entitled *Jewish Medical Ethics* to be short on medical ethical issues is unfortunate but in itself an instructive insight into the

---

8. Only the splinter Jewish sect of the Kararites and a minor citation by Rav Aha support the antimedical view.

state of the field in the early 1950s. Too much was yet to be. The revolutionary report of the ad hoc committee of the Harvard Medical School on brain death was almost a decade away when Jakobovits published his book. The first cardiac transplant was eight years away, and the abortion debate did not exist. Therefore it is not surprising that organ transplants rate but one inconclusive paragraph. Macro issues like societal allocation of scarce medical resources are not considered at all. The ethical problem of telling the truth to patients warrants a single sentence following a quote from 2 Kings 7.

When Jakobovits is forced to confront a medical ethical issue head-on, he often resorts to disappointing ambiguity. His treatment of euthanasia is instructive. Jakobovits cites the relevant sources as to the treatment of a *gosses*. The word comes from the Aramaic root word meaning the constriction of the chest and refers to a person considered to be no more than a couple of days away from death. The rabbinic position is that such a person must not be moved or even touched lest his or her life be prematurely ended by even the slightest contact, or in the more picturesque language of the Talmud cited by Jakobovits, "the matter can be compared with a flickering flame; as soon as one touches it, the light is extinguished" (1975: 122).

This would seem to imply a Jewish opposition to any act that might hasten a person's death, but Jakobovits also cites an important qualification to this teaching by the sixteenth-century Polish commentator to the *shulhan aruch*, Rabbi Moses Isserles from Krakow. Following earlier sources, he permits the removal of "anything causing a hindrance to the departure of the soul, such as a clattering noise near the patient's home (produced, for instance, by chopping wood) or salt on his tongue . . . , since such (action) involves no active [hastening of death], but only the removal of the impediment" (1975: 123; *Yoreh deah* 339).

Now when Jakobovits tries to explain how these contradictory Jewish teachings resolve the question of whether terminally ill patients can refuse or be refused medical treatment, he deals with the issue in the following way. If the patient is close to death, Jakobovits rules that *active euthanasia* is strictly prohibited (1975: 123). At the same time, he states, "Jewish law sanctions, and perhaps even demands, the withdrawal of any factor — whether extraneous to the patient himself or not — which may artificially delay his demise in the final phase. It might be argued that this modification implies the legality of expediting the death of an incurable patient in acute agony by withholding from him such

188

medicaments as sustain his continued life by unnatural means" (1975: 124). To this moral difficulty he responds, "Our sources advert only to cases in which death is expected to be imminent; it is, therefore, not altogether clear whether they would tolerate this moderate form of euthanasia, though that cannot be ruled out" (1975: 124). With this ambiguous comment, he leaves the issue hanging.

This is a good case in point. Jakobovits is solid on adducing relevant texts but disappointing in bringing out the moral implications of these texts. For example, he employs the distinction of active versus passive euthanasia (with Judaism forbidding the former and permitting the latter) but fails to differentiate the two. Thus there is no way to know whether any contemplated termination of care is more like silencing the woodchopper and therefore permitted by Jewish law or more like moving a *gosses* and thus prohibited.

Jakobovits was acutely aware of the time-bound limitations of his book and thus provided a supplemental chapter, "Recent Developments in Jewish Medical Ethics," in the 1975 edition. In this chapter Jakobovits addresses a variety of medical ethical issues, but unfortunately none for more than a page or two, and most in just a paragraph or two. This, for example, is the full treatment given to genetic engineering.

> Spare part surgery and genetic engineering may open a wonderful chapter in the history of healing. But without prior agreement on restraints and the strictest limitations, such mechanization of human life may also herald irretrievable disaster resulting from man's encroachment upon nature's preserves, from assessing human beings by their potential value as tool parts, sperm-donors or living incubators, and from replacing the matchless dignity of the human personality by test tubes, syringes and the soulless artificiality of computerized numbers. (1975: 266)

For a man who believes in the primacy of Jewish legal texts in the process of Jewish moral reasoning, this polemic is particularly sad. There is an utter absence of texts or Jewish sources that might illuminate the issue. At one time the respirator and heart-lung machine could surely have been criticized as leading to the "mechanization of human life" as well. Such comments tend to reinforce the theory that modern problems are too great a challenge for an ancient faith and legal corpus to confront.

What this chapter inadvertently reveals is a change that had occurred over the 15 years since the initial publication of *Jewish Medical Ethics*. During that time, the field of Jewish medical ethics was taken away from Rabbi Jakobovits and all other rabbis not engaged in full-time study and teaching of Jewish texts in the Yeshiva world. Deans of rabbinical seminaries and Orthodox academic institutions became the primary writers of responsa. Pulpit rabbis and communal leaders, even one with serious scholarly training like Jakobovits, had been surpassed. This change reduced creative Jewish thinkers like Jakobovits who lacked worldwide talmudic authority to the status of quoting the responsa of other rabbis rather than examining Jewish texts themselves.[9]

Jakobovits's new tentativeness, a reluctance to rule authoritatively on virtually any issue, reflects this new reality, which he himself delineates with grace and understanding. In this chapter, Jakobovits cites the responsa literature — the foundational texts are left to the authors of the responsa. This process is a modern example of the ongoing dynamic of Jewish law in which foundational texts become supplanted by commentaries that then become foundational texts for new commentaries. In the layering of interpretation of Jewish sources, all but the most learned are thrown off the track and reduced to the Jakobovitsian move of simply citing responsa while withholding personal judgment. One is left with a monotonous litany of "some authorities believe this . . . but other authorities believe that."

Another difficulty with Jakobovits's attempt to summarize recent developments in Jewish medical ethics is the growing diversity of opinion in these matters among non-Orthodox Jewish thinkers. As difficult as it is now to delineate a normative mainstream for Orthodox thinking in medical ethics, when the opinions of the liberal Jewish community are taken into account as well, consensus about the Jewish view of anything seems to collapse. Liberal Jewish thinkers have in the past two decades also analyzed these same Jewish sources and have often come to quite different conclusions about their normative thrust. Jakobovits does not give even a moment's notice to this interdenominational problem.

My own view is that Jewish sources are not completely elastic. It

---

9. This is particularly evident in his 1965 work for the Yeshiva University series *Studies in Torah Judaism* entitled *Jewish Law Faces Modern Problems,* in which he simply reviews the rulings of other *posekim,* usually without comment.

is possible, I believe — and in this I agree with Jakobovits — to save Jewish teachings in this field from the hopeless relativism that asserts that all opinions are Jewishly valid. Jewish sources reflect Jewish values, and those values permit and forbid, sanction and condemn, authorize and renounce. However, to make this claim for a normative mainstream in Jewish teachings about medical ethics, a philosophical critique must be provided. The critique will clarify the underlying values that drive Jewish legal rulings, and it will help articulate the reasons for the Jewish approach to medical ethical issues to non-Jewish thinkers.

III. Philosophical Critique

There must be a comprehensible way to explain to those outside the tradition just how Jewish moral decisions are made. This mode of explanation must neither distort the Jewish tradition in translating it into secular language nor pretend that a simple survey of Jewish sources can take the place of reasoned argument. This explanation of Jewish medical ethics, which we can call the philosophical translation of Jewish moral thinking, has not really been attempted, primarily because neither side has seen a need for it. Orthodox rabbis are generally not concerned about whether their rulings are understood by philosophers, and philosophers are generally not concerned about trying to understand the logic of rabbinical disputations and Jewish law.[10] I believe that this dialogue is crucial to both sides. Orthodox Judaism possesses a vast body of Jewish sources yet represents a small percentage of the Jewish world. Orthodox Jews must begin to understand that a world-renowned *posek* is known and respected in only a minutely small sphere. If Jewish moral reasoning and normative ethical thinking are to have any influence in the public debate, these Jewish scholars of the law must learn how to explain Jewish reasoning to people who are unfamiliar with it. Conversely, it is unconscionable that moral philosophers, who write about the supreme moral significance of human life and healing, be cavalierly

10. A good example of a philosopher who has both the knowledge of Jewish texts and the philosophical acumen to analyze their philosophical assumptions is Baruch Brody. His 1989 article on suicide and euthanasia is one of the best methodological attempts to translate Jewish sources philosophically without either distorting them or placing them outside the realm of philosophical critique.

indifferent to the tradition from which those values arose. Lacking a religious foundation, medical ethics must seek its resolutions in various forms of utilitarian or deontological schemes. These moral theories do not exhaust the moral choices real people face nor the choices that are theoretically possible. So the dialogue between Judaism and philosophy, which has had a long and spirited history, must now push forward into the realm of normative ethics.

As for Immanuel Jakobovits, despite his public service, his opposition to fundamentalism, and his great ecumenical efforts, it is not immediately evident that in his writings he truly intends secular philosophers (as opposed to the deans of the Yeshiva world) as his audience. Many of his essays were written as addresses to Christian clergy or to government officials. In these contexts Jakobovits's task was political or polemical and hardly scholarly. At his best he served as a kind of Jewish cultural historian to the British elites, who, it must be admitted, have never shown a great curiosity in matters Jewish. He reported on the Jewish tradition to the uninitiated in language that was faithful to its meaning, general, and perhaps incidentally compelling. Still, at other times he made eloquent appeals for "moral specialists" (undoubtedly meaning himself and other Orthodox rabbis) to prevent the "discretion of doctors" from being the sole determining guidance in the making of medical ethical decisions (1975: 256).

Only rarely does Jakobovits clearly intend to open a dialogue with secular philosophers and to present Jewish teachings as important not because they were authored by God through Moses and various rabbis, but because they contain good reasons, universalizable reasons, philosophically coherent reasons why someone, anyone, ought to concede that this or that Jewish teaching is not only quaint and eloquent but indeed true.

One important contribution of Jakobovits to the philosophical translation of Jewish moral reasoning is a distinction between human rights and human duties that he developed, all too briefly, in a 1976 address that is included in his collected essays (1989: 125-41). There Jakobovits delineates a critical element of Jewish moral reasoning. While much of modern ethical thinking speaks in the language of rights, Judaism, Jakobovits correctly asserts, speaks in the language of duties.

Now in Judaism we know of no intrinsic rights. Indeed there is no word for rights in the very language of the Hebrew Bible and of the classic sources of Jewish law. In the moral vocabulary of the Jewish discipline of life we speak of human duties, not of human rights, of obligations not entitlement. The Decalogue is a list of Ten Commandments not a Bill of Human Rights. In the charity legislation of the Bible, for instance, it is the rich man who is commanded to support the poor, not the poor man who has the right to demand support from the rich.

In Jewish law a doctor is obligated to come to the rescue of his stricken fellow-man and to perform any operation he considers essential for the life of the patient, even if the patient refuses his consent or prefers to die. Once again, the emphasis is on the physician's responsibility to heal, to offer service, more than on the patient's right to be treated. (1989: 128)

The distinction between an ethical system based on rights and an ethical system based upon duties is fundamental. One wishes that Jakobovits had dealt with this distinction and the philosophical issues raised by it in a systematic manner. What is the difference between, let us say, a person's right to private property and my duty not to steal what is his or hers? Ethical theory is full of debates on the differences between rights and duties, but there is no way to connect Judaism to that debate without a philosophically coherent idea of just how Judaism conceives of duties and whether it is actually true that Judaism has no notion of rights whatsoever. Jewish laws concerning private property and privacy offer prima facie evidence of rights language in Jewish law.

Still, Jakobovits is correct in saying that Jewish ethics turns on the fulcrum of duties rather than rights. Duties stem from a God who is believed to have dominion over all the universe and all that dwell in it, *ki kol ha'aretz li*, "for the whole earth is Mine, sayest the Lord." The nature of these duties precludes certain types of ethical arguments that are common in secular ethics. For example, arguments dependent on the premise that we own our bodies and therefore have a right to do with them what we wish to do are not acceptable. According to Judaism, God owns everything, including our bodies, and that ownership, based on Creation doctrines, when added to God's record of providential care, God's love and kindness to all creatures, and God's ethical will, establishes the moral force of our duties to do God's will.

The content of that will is a matter of intense dispute among the various branches of Judaism. What is not generally in dispute, however, are the underlying theological assumptions that establish our duty to do God's will in the world, however it is interpreted.

Rights theory, by contrast, arose historically in the context of the Enlightenment's attempt to overthrow the religiously based theories of the medieval period including the sinister and powerful theory of the divine right of kings. Rights theory, as developed by Locke and Hobbes particularly, establishes rights as personal prerogatives that derive from a state of nature that predates all historical religions and undermines their theocentric notion of duties. Rights are protections against the hostile incursions of others. Duties are the obligations that cause us to emerge from privatized lives and create morally significant communities.

In any event, these metaethical musings leave the concerns of Jakobovits far behind and address a new level of dialogue between Jewish thinkers and secular philosophers, a dialogue that has yet to begin in earnest.

IV. A Case in Point: Abortion

I think it useful to take a specific issue in medical ethics and consider it closely so that we can see just how Jakobovits's project fares when he tries to articulate the mode of Jewish ethical thinking to a larger audience. The topic I have chosen is abortion.

In Rabbi Jakobovits's earliest treatment of the abortion question he begins with a survey of abortion practices in Greek and Roman law, Catholic teaching, and civil legislation and finally moves to a survey of the rulings of Jewish law on the topic (1975: 170ff.). In his early work in the field he saw no need to offer a philosophical context for these rulings, but even then he showed that he was aware that Jewish law on abortion may appear obtuse at best and flatly contradictory at worst to even a sensitive non-Orthodox reader. The classic Jewish text is from *Mishnah Ohalot* 7:6.

> If a woman (even up to the moment of labor) has a (life-threatening) difficulty, one dismembers the embryo within her, removing it limb by limb (if necessary), because her life takes precedence over its life. But once a greater part (some say the head) has emerged (from the birth canal), it may not be harmed, for we do not set aside one life for another.

194

The problem with this text is that it does not explain why one may kill a fetus that threatens a mother's life during hard labor, but not kill a fetus that still threatens her life after its "greater part" has been delivered. One reasonable supposition is that Jewish law permitted the embryotomy because until birth the fetus was not yet considered a person, a bearer of moral rights. This is in fact the opinion of several authoritative rabbinic commentators.[11] In such a case, there is no conflict between persons, only a conflict between a woman and her "appendage."[12]

Yet, the birth of a fetus whose greater part has been delivered may still threaten the life of the mother. Judaism endorses self-defense against the attack of a "pursuer" (Leviticus 19:16; Deuteronomy 25:11-12; *sanhedrin* 73a, 74a), so why is the life of the fetus not forfeit for this reason? The Mishna asks that precise question and concludes that the woman is not at that point being pursued by the fetus but is being pursued "by the hands of Heaven" (*sanhedrin* 72b).

This talmudic answer does not clarify the situation. If the mother is being pursued "by the hands of Heaven" and not by the fetus, then why can the fetus be killed earlier, during hard labor? Jakobovits tries to explain the logic of the Talmud.

> But this consideration [that the fetus is a pursuer] does not arise before the main process of birth is complete, because we are not then dealing with two equal lives; or in the words of Rashi, "whatever has not come forth into the light of the world is not a human life." (1975: 184)

According to Jakobovits's understanding of this text, the fetus is a person, an object of full moral duties, when its major parts have emerged from the birth canal. At that point the Jewish principle "we do not set one life against another" applies. However, before the presentation of its "greater part" the fetus is not a full object of moral duties, not a fully juridical person, and therefore its destruction does not require the

---

11. Thus the medieval French commentator Rashi in his commentary to the talmudic tractate *sanhedrin* 72b. Also the Tosafists commentary to *niddah* 44b. The phrases used are quite explicit, *lav nefesh hu*, "(the fetus) is not a living soul," and *uhar yerech imo*, "the fetus is just an appendage of the mother."

12. The rabbinic belief that the fetus is not a person is consistent with a biblical text in Exodus (21:22; *sanhedrin* 84b).

strong claim of self-defense; when the fetus at this stage threatens the life of the mother, the inequality of its moral status vis-à-vis the mother is sufficient to justify its destruction.

Nevertheless, the great medieval authority Maimonides, and subsequent codifiers who relied upon him, revived the pursuer argument in his codification of *Mishnah Ohalot:*

> This too is a negative commandment: not to have compassion on the life of a pursuer. Therefore the sages ruled that when a woman has difficulty in labor one may dismember the embryo within her, either with drugs or with surgery, because he is like a pursuer seeking to kill her. But once the head has emerged, he may not be harmed, for we do not set aside one life for another. This is the natural course of the world.[13]

Jakobovits is obviously aware of the contradictions created by Maimonides's revival of the talmudically rejected pursuit argument:

> On the one hand, it relies on the "pursuer" argument to vindicate the operation; on the other, it dismisses its validity because nature, not the child, pursues the mother. Moreover, there seems to be a discrepancy between this ruling and the Mishnah which permits the deliberate sacrifice of the unborn child simply because its life is subordinated to that of the mother and not because she is being "pursued." (1975: 184-85)

Jakobovits tries to get Maimonides off the hook by citing rabbinic authorities, for example, Rabbi Yair Bacharach, who wrote that even though the fetus is not a person, it is enough like a person to make its destruction a moral, if not a capital, offense, and thus the pursuit argument is needed to justify killing it (*Hovot Yair* #31; Jakobovits 1975: 185 n. 159). Second, Jakobovits cites Rabbi Ezekiel Landau that one does not kill a dying person without good cause, even though the killing of a dying person is also not a capital crime, and thus pursuit is needed to bolster the lack of fetal personhood.[14] And finally Jakobovits offers

13. *Mishnah Torah*, "*hilchot rotzeiach*" (the laws of the murderer) 1:9 and in the *Shulhan Aruch* of Rabbi Yosef Karo, *hoschen mishpat* cdxxv.2.
14. *noday beyehuda* pt. ii, *chosen mishpat* #59. Jakobovits 1975: 185 nn. 161-62.

his own reasoning, that Maimonides needed the pursuit argument because after the birth process had begun but before the final stages of labor had commenced, the fetus moved into a new status, not yet person, but not any longer merely an appendage of the mother (1975: 185-86).

However needed the pursuit argument may be, the fact remains that the Talmud considered it and rejected it, and Maimonides's restoration of this argument in his code is a clear contradiction of the earlier rabbinic tradition. Maimonides does couch his description of the fetal threat to the mother's life by saying that the fetus is *k'rodef*, "like a pursuer," and thus there is room to save the integrity of the talmudic ruling. The self-defense claim is critical to the Jewish moral logic on the abortion question. It is not needed to explain why a fetus may be killed when it threatens the life of the mother, but rather is needed to explain why the fetus may *not* be killed when it does *not* pose a threat to the life of the mother.

Maimonides foresaw, and Jakobovits does not see this, that if the fetus is not a person, and if the pursuit in dangerous pregnancies is "from Heaven" and not from the fetus, there is no reason for Jewish law to oppose abortion even when the mother's life is not at risk. If the fetus is just "an appendage of the mother," what moral issues are at stake in its destruction? And yet the Jewish legal tradition has consistently ruled that only therapeutic abortions, abortions where the life or health of the mother is at risk, are permissible.

In fact, Jewish law never was forced to consider arguments for purely elective abortions until our own time, and Jewish sources on abortion are not in total agreement about the moral status of the fetus.[15]

---

15. Indeed, the same Rashi who authored *lav nefesh hu*, "the fetus is not a person," states in his commentary to *sanhedrin* 85b that one who kidnaps a pregnant woman is culpable for not one but two kidnappings, the mother and the fetus! Furthermore, the talmudic tractate *arachin* 7a commands that medical implements be carried (in violation of Sabbath law) to attempt the delivery of a fetus from a woman who is already dead. In a revealing nonlegal passage in the Talmud, the Emperor Antoninus was said to have engaged Rabbi Judah ha-Nasi in a debate over when the soul enters the body. The rabbi answered "from birth," and the emperor argued that it entered at the time of conception. He asks the rabbi, "Meat cannot remain three days without spoiling and you say the soul which preserves the body only enters at birth?" Remarkably, this great Jewish sage is convinced by the Roman emperor's argument. Finally, there is the verse from Job, "From the womb I have known thee." These texts seem to establish that there was a strong tradition in Judaism that treated the fetus as if it were a person, despite Rashi's comments. Maimonides was aware of this inconsistent tradition, and he rectified it

In a later essay written in 1967 and revised in 1973 Jakobovits attempts his most ambitious philosophical translation of Jewish sources on abortion.[16] He writes,

> The judgement that is required here, while it must be based on medical evidence, is clearly of a moral nature. The decision on whether, and under what circumstances, it is right to destroy a germinating human life depends on the assessment and weighing of values, on determining the title to life in any given case. Such value judgments are entirely outside the province of medical science. . . . Such judgments pose essentially a moral, not a medical problem. (1989: 348)

He offers a judgment that Judaism has indeed embodied a system of ethics — a definition of moral values. In what one must presume is a blast aimed at Kantian demands for autonomous not heteronomous ethics he defends his version of heteronomy.

> In the Jewish view, the human conscience is meant to enforce laws, not to make them. Right and wrong, good and evil, are absolute values which transcend the capricious variations of time, place and environment, just as they defy definition by relation to human intuition or expediency. These values, Judaism teaches, derive their validity from the Divine revelation at Mount Sinai, as expounded and developed by sages faithful to, and authorized by, its writ. (1989: 349)

He believes that "for a definition of these values, one must look to the vast and complex corpus of Jewish law, the authentic expression of all Jewish religious and moral thought" (1989: 349). This is a serious systematic mistake. Jewish law never intended to define Jewish values in any coherent philosophical sense. There is no catechism of values, no systematic theology stating Jewish foundational values or those values derived from them. Jewish law is not presented in a systematic

---

brilliantly by his inclusion of the pursuer argument. Reform rabbis like Balfour Brickner and Bernard Zlotowitz have consistently maintained that the Orthodox rabbinate has distorted the teachings of Judaism on abortion, teachings that in their view should support a woman's right to choose an abortion (Brickner 1978). See also the exchange between Brickner and Bleich in *Sh'ma* (1985).

16. "Jewish Views on Abortion" can be found in Walbert and Butler 1973 and Jakobovits 1989.

philosophical schema. Values are instantiated in Jewish law, not defined by it. Those values must be found out by complex and always tenuous exegesis. This is the central methodological problem that any Orthodox Jewish thinker must surmount in order to bring the insights of the Jewish legal tradition into dialogue with the philosophically literate secular world. Further, the selection of which sages are authorized to interpret these values to the world is a matter of intense debate even among religious Jews.

Jakobovits moves to his philosophical translation of Jewish sources on abortion in a section of this essay entitled "Moral and Social Considerations." I want to consider it closely, for it is a rare example in Jakobovits's work of his venturing out beyond an archival summary of Jewish sources into the battlefield of normative ethical theory where talmudic citations do not suffice to convince.

First, Jakobovits considers the argument that Jewish laws and other restrictive abortion laws are cruel. To this objection he offers the following response:

> There is, inevitably, some element of cruelty in most laws. To a person who has spent his last cent before the tax bill arrives, the income tax laws are unquestionably "cruel"; and to a man passionately in love with a married woman the adultery laws must appear "barbaric". Even more universally harsh are the military draft regulations which expose young men to acute danger and their families to great anguish and hardship. All these "cruelties" are surely no valid reason for changing those laws. No civilized society could survive without laws which occasionally cause some suffering for individuals. Nor can any public moral standards be maintained without strictly enforced regulations calling for extreme restraints and sacrifices in some cases. If the criterion for the legitimacy of laws were the complete absence of "cruel" effects, we should abolish or drastically liberalize not only our abortion laws, but our statutes on marriage, narcotics, homosexuality, suicide, euthanasia, and numerous other matters, which inevitably result in personal anguish from time to time. (1989: 354)

Jakobovits wants us to disregard the cruel consequences of a law because all laws produce some cruel consequences. But this argument is clearly false for a variety of evident reasons:

1. Cruel consequences are indeed one of the ways we determine

that some laws are unjust. Are we to bear the cruelty of legalized slavery or legalized genocide simply because all laws have some cruel consequences? The laws against homosexuals, against persons deciding whether or not to continue medical treatment, or against those who wish to use drugs legally, are all subject to serious charges of cruelty as well as unjustified paternalism. Furthermore, this argument relates only to our judgment of abortion laws, not to the morality of abortion itself, which is the question at issue here.

2. His examples are not clearly examples of cruelty. The angst of a taxpayer caught short of funds could not reasonably be called a cruel consequence of the tax laws if the person is a profligate spendthrift, but if the taxpayer is a victimized poor person being further oppressed by a confiscatory taxing authority, then it would be cruel and cast doubt on the morality of the tax laws. Similarly, it is clear that the moral case for the draft must be made and cannot be assumed.

Jakobovits's attempt to disregard consequentialist arguments fails, but he does realize that the key question is not the effect of the laws, but rather the moral justification for their existence. "It remains to be demonstrated," Jakobovits acknowledges, "that the restrictions on abortion are morally sound enough and sufficiently important to the public welfare to outweigh the consequential hardships in individual cases" (1989: 354).

What arguments does he put forward to support the thesis that restrictions on abortion are morally sound, important to the public welfare, and outweigh the consequential hardships in individual cases? This is hard to know. Jakobovits continues:

> What the fuming editorials and harrowing documentaries on the abortion problem do not show are pictures of radiant mothers fondling perfectly healthy children who would never have been alive if their parents had been permitted to resort to abortion in moments of despair. . . . Some children may be born unwanted, but there are few unwanted children aged five or ten years. (1989: 354-55)

It is hard to know just what Jakobovits is asserting here. Perhaps it is something like, "Abortion ought to be morally and legally proscribed because upon experiencing motherhood the woman will change her mind and love and accept the child." If this is what he means, he brings not a single shred of evidence to support this assertion. Indeed, the statement that there are no unwanted children aged five or ten is obviously and tragically wrong.

And the question remains, How does the variable and subjective attitude of pregnant women toward their fetuses establish the moral grounds for or against abortion? Jakobovits gives us no help with this. He then argues that a liberalizing of the laws would increase the number of abortions, but if abortion is morally justifiable, then these statistics are not relevant.

Finally, Jakobovits admits that we cannot resolve the morality of abortion based on numbers; he then proceeds to a Jewish value that he quotes from the Talmud, "He who saves one life is as if he saved an entire world."[17] On the basis of this talmudic dictum, Jakobovits considers the abortion of deformed fetuses and also those conceived by rape or incest as violations of the sanctity-of-life principle.

As for deformed fetuses or fetuses suspected of being deformed, he states, "So long as the sanctity of life is recognized as inviolable, the cure for suffering cannot be abortion before birth, any more than murder (whether in the form of euthanasia or suicide) after birth. The only legitimate relief in such cases is for society to assume the burdens which the individual family can no longer bear" (1989: 355).

As for pregnancies caused by rape, Jakobovits asserts that "the circumstances of such a conception can have little bearing on the child's title to life, and in the absence of any well-grounded challenge to this title there cannot be any moral justification for an abortion" (1989: 356). Similarly for pregnancies resulting from incest, adultery, or otherwise illegitimate relations Jakobovits opposes abortion as a morally justified act. In these cases the child is considered a *mamzer* in Jewish law and is severely stigmatized by a multitude of prohibitions and reduced status in the Jewish community. Jakobovits defends this stigmatization of innocent children as constituting a laudable deterrent to immoral behavior in the adult community, and as a legitimate consequence of parental responsibility,

> Strict abortion laws, ruling out the post facto "correction" of rash
> acts, compel people to think twice *before* they recklessly embark on
> illicit or irresponsible adventures liable to inflict lifelong suffering or

17. Mishna in tractate *sanhedrin* 4:5 and Maimonides *Mishna Torah* "hilchot *yesodei ha-torah*" 5:5.

infamy on their progeny. To eliminate the scourge of illegitimate children, more self-discipline to prevent their conception is required, not more freedom to destroy them in the womb. (1989: 357-58)

Neither the conditions causing the pregnancy nor the condition of the fetus seems to affect the moral judgment on abortion made by Jakobovits.

However, there are a multitude of problems with this the most serious argument adduced by Jakobovits.

1. Why are we to assume that the fetus is able to claim defense under the sanctity-of-life principle? The point at issue is precisely whether the fetus is a bearer of moral rights like other human persons, and so one cannot use the moral claims of acknowledged persons to cover the fetus without begging the question at issue. Some arguments must be provided to defend fetal personhood, and Jakobovits gives us no such argument.

Given Rashi's commentary that the fetus is not a person (*nefesh*), there is, as we have remarked, good reason to use the Jewish tradition to support and not condemn elective abortions. Jakobovits concludes, for reasons never delineated, that the killing of a fetus, though not a capital crime, is still a severe moral offense.

But many liberal rabbis have concluded that abortion is neither murder nor a serious moral offense. We are forced to conclude that both the facts of fetal development and the teachings of Jewish law give ample evidence to both sides of the debate about fetal personhood.

2. It does seem, at the very least, inconsistent for Jakobovits to claim that the sanctity-of-life principle protects a fetus from being killed but does not protect a fetus from being discriminated against as the product of an incestuous union simply for the sake of public moral edification. If these are innocent beings who ought not be killed unjustifiably because of their innocence, then surely they ought not be stigmatized by reason of that same innocence. The willingness to defend such truly cruel laws, which prevent such children from marrying anyone but another *mamzer*, from praying in a synagogue, or from being buried in a Jewish cemetery while at the same time claiming to protect their infinite value is difficult to comprehend even for someone schooled in Orthodox casuistry.

3. Even more astounding is Jakobovits's refusal to allow abortion in cases of rape. The Jewish legal tradition has a long tradition of allowing therapeutic abortions not only to save the mother's life but to

protect her psychological well-being. Rabbi Jacob Emden, a prominent German *posek* of the eighteenth century, ruled that a pregnancy caused by an adulterous union could be allowed to save the woman from the "great pain" of such an embarrassing pregnancy (*she'elat yavetz* #43). Rabbi Ben Zion Meir Ha Uziel permitted an abortion to save a pregnant woman from becoming deaf in both her ears due to the pregnancy. Rabbi Yechiel Weinberg, a Swiss rabbi, in 1966 permitted an abortion for a woman who contracted German measles during pregnancy. Rabbi Eliezer Waldenberg allowed the abortion of even a seventh-month Tay-Sachs fetus as therapeutic. Rabbi Issar Unterman also included extreme mental anguish as grounds for declaring an abortion to be therapeutic. Forcing a rape victim to endure a double ignominy stretched out over nine months and then to negotiate with the rapist for care of the child is not a normative Jewish position.

On a philosophical level, Jakobovits wrongly assumes that in the absence of any well-grounded challenge to the fetus's right to life abortion in such cases cannot be morally justified. In fact without a well-grounded defense of the fetus's right to life abortions in such cases cannot be morally condemned either! Rabbi Jakobovits does not give us any good reasons for considering a fetus a bearer of moral rights, and thus his use of the sanctity-of-life argument fails to convince.

Having rejected all other reasons to justify abortions, Jakobovits finally comes to the issue of protecting the mother's safety through therapeutic abortions. Because the Jewish legal tradition has endorsed therapeutic abortions from its beginning, it is not surprising to find Jakobovits also philosophically predisposed to favoring the mother in such an ultimate conflict of rights.

> Such a threat to the mother need not be either immediate or absolutely certain. Even a remote risk of life involves all the life-saving concessions of Jewish law, provided the fear of such a risk is genuine and confirmed by the most competent medical opinions. Hence, Jewish law would regard it as an indefensible desecration of human life to allow a mother to perish in order to save her unborn child. (1989: 358)

The reason for this conclusion is of course the rabbinic view of the difference in the status of the fetus and the mother, which allows Jakobovits morally to prefer the life of the mother. That differential can be maintained in the Talmud by one citation from a recognized authority, but that will not suffice if Jakobovits intends a philosophical defense of the Jewish position.

Jakobovits tries to skirt this issue by arguing for a divine ascription of value to human life.

> In the view of Judaism, all human rights, and their priorities, derive solely from their conferment upon man by his Creator. By this criterion, as defined in the Bible, the rights of the mother and her unborn child are distinctly unequal, since the capital guilt of murder takes effect only if the victim is a born viable person. This recognition does not imply that the destruction of a fetus is not a very grave offense against the sanctity of human life, but only that it is not technically murder. (1989: 358)

The proven viability of the mother seems to be the decisive point here in giving her priority over the fetus who is of unproven viability. Taken as a philosophical argument, this opens up an interesting train of thought. If both will die but one can live if the other is killed, we are told to prefer the one of proven viability.

This seems to be adequate reasoning, but we soon see that viability is a slippery concept. First, it varies as the state of medical science increases. Further, a woman with uterine cancer who has an abortion so as to proceed with radiation treatments that may not save her life would be less viable than her healthy fetus, whose birth must be purchased at her certain death. Therefore we cannot conclude that the fetus will always be less viable than the mother (particularly after the first trimester), and so any arguments based on differences of status through viability are dubious at best.

If, on the other hand, we are to accept the difference in status as the result of God's decree, how do we reconcile that decree with the sanctity-of-life principle in which all life is of infinite value and the fetus is clearly an instance of human life?

V. Conclusion

Medical ethical problems have forced religious thinkers to enter the realm of public discourse, what Richard Neuhaus has called "the naked public square," and try to bring moral reasoning with religious foundations into a world that seems to resist all values and moral critique. Medical ethics issues strike at the core of religious values and prompt urgent appeals to the religious traditions for moral guidance. To his great credit, Rabbi Immanuel Jakobovits understands this, and his concern for the relevance of Jewish law to the problems of modern life led him to discover and nurture in its infancy the field of Jewish medical ethics.

Orthodox rabbis have been ruling on such matters for thousands of years, but their rulings were crafted for a homogeneous community. In the harsh but invigorating winds of the democratic secularism that defines the debate in America and England, the rulings of an Orthodox rabbi carry much less weight. Jakobovits understood this and tried to articulate Jewish laws to non-Orthodox Jews and to Christians. The question we must ask is whether or not he succeeds.

On one level he fails because he cannot and does not engage in a systematic explication of the values and principles at work in the formation of Jewish law. Thus, most of the dynamic and the conclusions of that law remain inaccessible to all but the sympathetic Orthodox Jewish reader. What he does do with mastery is collect the primary sources and describe the legal precedents and normative conclusions of that legal tradition. He does not, however, give a non-Orthodox Jew good reasons to consider this tradition the embodiment of moral truth. His excursus into philosophical issues is often crude, attenuated, and utterly unconvincing. Immanuel Jakobovits is a fine rabbi and master of Jewish law but, in my view, he did not succeed in the task of philosophical translation that alone will facilitate the dialogue between Judaism and the secular world.

Furthermore, his hermeneutic that truth is given to Moses and explicated by authoritative sages is belied by his own method.[18] The bitter divisions among respected Orthodox sages destroy the assertion that truth, even revealed truth, is black and white and manifest in the mouths of modern rabbis singed with the smoke of Sinai.

---

18. He argues that the dictates of Jewish law forbid abortion for pregnancies caused by rape or incest or to avoid the birth of a deformed infant, yet in a postscript to his article on abortion he cites the rulings of the Chief Rabbi of Jerusalem that contradict these judgments and allow abortions in precisely those cases! Rabbi Eliezer Waldenberg, *Tzitz Eliezer*, pt. 7, #41; pt. 9, #51; Jakobovits 1989: 359n.53.

Can any Jewish thinker pull this off? Can anyone speak out of the authentic sources of Judaism while also speaking in a voice that can make Jewish values accessible and compelling to those who are not predisposed to consider those sources morally definitive?

I think the project of Jewish medical ethics is possible and necessary for the edification of the public debate, and it must proceed and engage an even deeper dialogue with philosophers and physicians doing this work. All moral judgments emerge from a particular tradition of moral discourse, and, however abstruse, Judaism is one of those grounds of value that has formed the West and continues to serve as a standard against which the society can be measured and its moral vacuousness exposed.

Those who seek to do Jewish medical ethics, however, must attend to several concerns:

1. *Jewish law must be seen as a product of both history and Sinai.* Revelation stands behind the Jewish laws, but they are and were written by people who live and lived in a certain historical context. Jewish thinkers must see the Jewish legal tradition not as the unalloyed speech of God but as the attempts of fallible human beings to cope with the progressive and ongoing nature of God's revelation to the Jewish people about the way they should live in the world. This enables a critique of even authoritative rabbis as they here succeed and there fail in offering a coherent approach to these ethical problems.

2. *Philosophy must be seen as a tool not an antagonist in the project of making God's will known to us.* The highest and most golden ages of both Christianity and Judaism were the moments when the faculties of the mind joined with the gifts of the spirit in speaking the truth to the world. Jakobovits chose two good models in Maimonides and Hirsch, both the products of the highest philosophical traditions of their time. A Jewish legal tradition that is impenetrable to outsiders and filled with inconsistencies and unexamined premises is of no value to Jews, Christians, or secularists. The authority of religious pronouncements must be buttressed by their inherent reasonableness, not just by some appeal to lightning and thunder. It is the first principles that need to be undergirded and justified by faith in God's revelation, not the details of how those principles work themselves out in normative ethical judgments.

The way Jakobovits should have defended the Jewish position on abortion, in my judgment, was not to venture into consequentialist arguments about how we must accept a little cruelty in our laws to avoid

206

anarchy, or accept restrictive abortion laws to avoid rampaging moral lassitude (both highly dubious and ultimately non-Jewish arguments), but rather to examine carefully the Jewish belief in the sanctity of life.

This value is not absolute as he says, but it is very strong and strong enough to protect innocent life that poses no threat to the mother. The Jewish values of the sanctity of life and the divine ownership of our bodies, when combined with the Jewish belief that we are morally bound to each other by duties that flow from God through natural law and not by rights that flow from governments enacting state laws, will generate, I believe, a philosophically coherent defense of the Jewish views on abortion.

Only the primal values require revelation as their source and justification. After that, how these values work in protecting fetuses, deformed children, dying persons, poor people, and all those who sleep in the dust will be wholly rational, philosophically coherent, and morally uplifting. If the task is undertaken with reason and faith, it will bring us to the doing of justice, the love of mercy, and the humble walking with our God.

To this ancient and morally profound system let our critics bring their calls for private rights and selfish prerogatives and individual freedoms. Let them try to build communities one isolated monad at a time. Let them try to find virtue as one person sits under a fig tree, alone, and surrounded by the protections of the modern state, which assure at one and the same time utter defense from the incursions of others and also utter loneliness and isolation from all others — made also in the image of God. As for us, we shall heal and try to teach God's Torah of healing to all who are sick and will listen.

References

Abramson, Glenda, ed. 1989. *Blackwell Companion to Jewish Culture.* Oxford, England: Basil Blackwell.

Bleich, J. David. 1977, 1983. *Contemporary Halakhic Problems.* 2 vols. Hoboken, N.J.: KTAV Publishing and Yeshiva University Press.

———. 1981. *Judaism and Healing.* Hoboken, N.J.: KTAV Publishing.

———. 1985. "A Critique of Brickner on Abortion." *Sh'ma* 5 (January 10).

Brickner, Balfour. 1978, "Judaism and Abortion." In *Contemporary Jewish Ethics,* ed. Menachem Marc Kellner, 279-83. New York: Sanhedrin Press.

Brickner, Balfour. 1985. "A Critique of Bleich on Abortion." *Sh'ma* 5 (January 10).

Brody, Baruch. 1972. *Abortion and the Sanctity of Human Life: A Philosophical View.* Cambridge, Mass.: MIT Press.

———. 1983. "The Use of Halakhic Material in Discussions of Medical Ethics." *Journal of Medicine and Philosophy* 8: 317-28.

———. 1988. *Life and Death Decision-Making.* New York: Oxford University Press.

———. 1989. "A Historical Introduction to Jewish Casuistry on Suicide and Euthanasia." In *Suicide and Euthanasia,* ed. Baruch Brody, 39-75. Dordrecht: Kluwer Academic Publishers.

Fackenheim, Emil. 1973. *Encounters between Judaism and Modern Philosophy.* New York: Basic Books.

Fein, Leonard, ed. 1987, "A *Moment* Interview with Immanuel Jakobovits, Chief Rabbi of England." In *Jewish Possibilities: The Best of* Moment *Magazine.* Northvale, N.J.: Jason Aaronson.

Feldman, David. 1968. *Birth Control in Jewish Law.* New York: New York University Press.

Jakobovits, Immanuel. [1959] 1975. *Jewish Medical Ethics: A Comparative and Historical Study of the Jewish Religious Attitudes to Medicine and Its Practice.* 4th ed. rev. and enl. New York: Bloch Publishing.

———. 1963. *Hospital Compendium: A Guide to Jewish Moral and Religious Principles in Hospital Practice.* New York: Commission on Synagogue Relations of the Federation of Jewish Philanthropies.

———. 1965. *Jewish Law Faces Modern Problems: Some Questions and Answers Compiled and Reviewed.* New York: Yeshiva University.

———. 1966. *Journal of a Rabbi.* New York: Living Books.

———. 1989. *The Timely and the Timeless: Jews, Judaism and Society in a Storm-tossed Decade.* New York: Bloch Publishing.

Rosner, Fred. 1972. *Modern Medicine and Jewish Law.* New York: Bloch Publishing for Yeshiva University Press.

———. 1986. *Modern Medicine and Jewish Ethics.* New York: KTAV Publishing and Yeshiva University Press.

Rosner, Fred, and J. David Bleich. 1979. *Jewish Bioethics.* New York: Sanhedrin Press.

Tendler, Moshe. 1968. "Medical Ethics and Torah Morality." *Tradition* (Spring).

Walbert, David F., and J. Douglas Butler. 1973. *Abortion, Society, and the Law.* Cleveland: Press of Case Western Reserve University.

Wolf, Arnold. 1976. "Judaism on Medicine." *Yale Journal of Biology and Medicine* 49: 385-89.

ON BERNARD HÄRING

Construing Medical Ethics Theologically

RON P. HAMEL

IN THE fall of 1939, a 27-year-old German from the town of Böttingen was conscripted into Hitler's army along with many other young men. Bernard Häring, who had been ordained a Catholic priest in the Redemptorist Order a few months earlier, was assigned to serve as a medic. He had been slated to teach moral theology in the Redemptorist seminary when the orders arrived; at the request of his superiors, he received a nine-month deferral. During those months of teaching, Häring conceived and outlined a three-volume work in moral theology. *The Law of Christ* would be published (in German) in 1954 and become a seminal work in the field. But before he actually undertook the writing of the book, Häring served for five years — ministering as a medic (and illegally as a priest) not only to German troops but also to Russian soldiers and civilians and to segments of the Polish population. These were formative years for Häring. Among other things, his war experiences led him to question the moral theology he had learned as a seminary student. He gradually came to see it as abstract, legalistic, rigid, and out of touch with the complexities of ordinary life. Häring writes:

> Like most priests at that time, I was trained in a rather strict understanding of law and of obedience to law. The turmoil of those years had a liberating effect on me. . . .
>
> Looking back, I see the difficult experiences of the war as a hard school for discovering the unique value of freedom of conscience, the

right meaning of responsibility and responsible obedience, as well as a more mature approach to law, including church law. (1976a: 76, 67)

The impact of Häring's war experiences on his understanding of Christian moral life has been felt throughout the Roman Catholic world and beyond. No contemporary figure has had greater influence on the reshaping of Catholic moral theology, particularly through his major work for clergy and laity, *The Law of Christ* (1961, 1963a, 1966), translated into at least 11 languages. American Catholic theologian Charles Curran gave this assessment: "Häring's work stands as the most creative and important accomplishment in moral theology in this century, and the case could be made that it is the most original and significant contribution in the recent history of the discipline of moral theology" (1982: 145). Since 1954, Häring has published more than 65 books, a second three-volume work on fundamental moral theology, and numerous articles. Their topics range from fundamental moral theology, issues in Christian life and spirituality, and church and sacraments, to particular areas of moral theology such as marriage and the family, the Christian use of violence, and medical ethics.

Little of this corpus is devoted to medical ethics. What is consists for the most part of two books, *Medical Ethics* (1973a) and *Ethics of Manipulation* (1976b), chapters in both of his three-volume works in moral theology, and several essays. The majority of this work was done in the early to mid-1970s; he has written little on the subject since. Most of his conclusions on issues would probably be considered mainstream among Roman Catholic ethicists today (though many were not when first proposed). Some would undoubtedly be viewed as conservative, both within and outside of the Catholic tradition. It cannot be said that Häring's work is the most fully articulated and systematically reasoned, with regard to either methodology or the moral assessment of specific biomedical developments. What then commends it for consideration?

Häring's actual and potential contribution to medical ethics can be appreciated only if his work is understood within two contexts — Roman Catholic moral theology and medical ethics, and contemporary American medical ethics. With regard to the former, Häring's significance lies in a reinterpretation of Christian moral life that differs substantially from the one dominant in Catholicism since the mid-sixteenth century. The older approach to moral theology, typically taken in standard textbooks used in seminaries, tended to be highly philosophical (employing a form of natural law reasoning), concerned with the application of universal and unchanging principles to particular actions and situations in a deductive manner, preoccupied with judgments of the rightness or wrongness of actions, committed to the integrity of biological processes in a virtually absolute way, and divorced from concrete human experience. The result was not only a rigid, fairly negative morality of law and obedience, but one that barely reflected the nature of Christian existence as depicted in the Christian scriptures. A similar treatment of medical issues characterized the manuals of moral theology from the mid-sixteenth century on as well as the textbooks of medical ethics developed in Europe in the latter part of the nineteenth and first half of the twentieth centuries and in the United States in the 1940s and 1950s.[1]

The winds began to shift in the early years of the twentieth century, when a number of European moral theologians began to reinterpret and reformulate Catholic moral theology.[2] Inspired by their work and his own experiences, Häring, in the mid-1950s and after, carried the effort forward in a decisive manner. Initiatives by other moral theologians followed, particularly after the Second Vatican Council. Eventually, the reorientation that was occurring in fundamental moral theology began to take hold in medical morality as well. Conclusions that had been reached on the basis of the older methodology were questioned, as was the methodology itself. Bernard Häring played an important role in this process. The resulting medical ethics was very different in nature and scope from that propounded in standard Catholic medical moral textbooks.

Häring's work also contrasts sharply with the medical ethics that has developed in the United States. While much of his writing in the area occurred during formative years in the development of U.S. medical ethics, each developed in very different directions. When the American bioethics movement began in the 1960s it was very much influenced by religious approaches. But over the past 20 years American bioethics has become increasingly secularized, in part because ethicists wanted it to

---

1. The most prominent of the medical moral textbooks to originate in this country are Edwin Healy's *Medical Ethics* (1956); Gerald A. Kelly's *Medico-Moral Problems* (1958); John Kenny's *Principles of Medical Ethics* (1952); Charles McFadden's *Medical Ethics* ([1949] 1961); and Thomas O'Donnell's *Morals in Medicine* (1956).

2. Among the most notable of these moral theologians were Otto Schilling (*Handbuch der Moraltheologie* [1934]; *Die Verwirklichung der Nachfolge Christi* [1935-36]) and Gérard Gilleman (*Le primat de la charité en théologie morale* [1952]).

be widely relevant in a pluralistic society. Philosophical and legal influences now dominate and define the field and shape discourse. By and large it is characterized by the explication and subsequent application to cases of the two major ethical theories (deontology and teleology) and four principles (respect for autonomy, beneficence, nonmaleficence, and justice) (see, for example, Beauchamp and Childress 1979). The application of principles to cases has become paradigmatic of medical ethics in the United States. This standard "principles approach," combined with the strong influence of traditional American liberal values and modes of thinking, has made medical ethics in the United States a dilemma-oriented, problem-solving, deductive, rationalistic, individualistic, and rights-focused enterprise. Consequently, other considerations (for example, community and the common good, duties and responsibilities) and ultimate questions (for example, the nature and purpose of life and the meaning of suffering) are neglected. Häring's medical ethics is by no means the corrective to the U.S. model, but it does offer a contrast. Perhaps its greatest strength (which some might well consider its greatest weakness) is that it does medical ethics theologically and in doing so offers an integral, theologically grounded understanding of fundamental human questions. Thus Häring's medical ethics provides a richer context for assessing developments in medicine and science.

In this essay, I delineate some of the main aspects of Häring's fundamental moral theology on which his medical ethics is based. Then I discuss a number of the major constitutive elements of his medical ethics that distinguish it from traditional Roman Catholic and standard U.S. models. Because it is principally these constitutive, methodological dimensions that differentiate Häring's approach, they will be the exclusive focus of discussion. Virtually no attention will be given to his handling of specific issues.

Häring's Reorientation of Catholic Moral Theology

A Religious and Biblically Informed Interpretation of Moral Life

In an oft-cited article that appeared some years ago, James Gustafson chided religious ethicists working in medical ethics for abandoning their responsibility to do Christian ethics theologically. "The relation of their moral discourse to any specific theological principles," he writes, "or even to a definable religious outlook is opaque" (Gustafson 1978: 386). More recently, Leon Kass, reflecting on the current mode of ethical reflection, observed: "Perhaps for the sake of getting a broader hearing, perhaps not to profane sacred teachings or to preserve a separation between the things of God and the things of Caesar, most religious ethicists entering the public practice of ethics leave their special insights at the door and talk about 'deontological vs. consequentialist,' 'autonomy vs. paternalism,' 'justice vs. utility,' just like everybody else" (Kass 1990: 6-7).

This charge cannot be leveled at Häring. From the outset he believed that although religion and morality are autonomous realities, for the Christian they are intimately related. Häring's vital interest in articulating a religious ethics grew out of his intense concern over the virtual divorce of Catholic natural law morality from its religious sources — which he considered to be not only a serious impoverishment but also a deviation from the biblical tradition.

An ethic can be religious for Häring only if it possesses the same structure as religion itself. His phenomenological analysis of religion led him to conclude that religion is essentially personal, dialogical, and responsive.[3] It involves a personal, transcendent Thou advancing toward the individual in self-disclosure and inviting the person into relationship, and the believing, trusting, loving, and worshipping response of the person. The essence of religion is word-response, fellowship between the divine and the human. This is what Häring calls a "sacral ethic."

The relationship between religion and morality springs from the recognition of the sacred Thou as Supreme Value and as the ground of all particular values. If moral values are ultimately grounded in the holy, so then is the obligation they impose upon human beings for respect. Hence to respond to moral values is also to respond to the value of the sacred that grounds them. Recognition of the relationship between moral values and the sacred is a stance of faith, an intuition of the heart (1963b: 47-50, 55-84). Hence, though each has its distinct character, its particular object of concern, and its unique requirements,

---

3. Häring gives systematic attention to the relationship of religion and morality in his dissertation, *Das Heilige und Das Gute. Religion und Sittlichkeit in ihrem gegenseitigen Bezug,* published in 1950. References in this essay are to the French translation: *Le sacré et le bien* (1963b). A brief discussion also occurs in *The Law of Christ* (1961: 35-49).

religion and morality are not mutually exclusive and in fact are related in their depths.

Both the self-disclosure of the holy and the response of the human are mediated. For Christians, Jesus Christ is the preeminent self-manifestation of the sacred as well as of the human response of faith, obedient love, and worship. Both sides of the dialogue are embodied in him, and it is primarily in and through him that the Christian encounters and responds to the sacred. Although he is the primordial revelation of God, he is not the sole one. All creation is revelatory, and particularly human beings. Thus response to these forms of revelation is also indirectly response to the sacred. Here too Jesus Christ is paradigmatic. Community with and faithful obedience to the Godhead results in redeeming love for fellow humans. Given all of this, Häring considers a morality based on discipleship to Christ to be the one that best integrates and expresses the constitutive elements of a religious ethic (1963b: 246-63).

Any ethic not founded on fellowship with the sacred and not ultimately a response to the sacred cannot be, for Häring, a religious ethic (1963b: 195-243; 1961: 39-42). This would include conceptions of ethics in which the human is both the ground and goal of all moral obligation and activity. Systems that focus on human happiness, self-perfection, salvation, or eternal beatitude do not qualify as religious ethics. Häring unequivocally rejects the human person and human self-perfection as the ultimate basis of a religious ethic, though he does not negate or minimize their significance. A true religious ethic has as its ultimate reference the sacred. Though moral activity is directed to the needs and dignity of human beings and to created reality, it is at the same time a response to the sacred who is present in and through these. Just as people and nature are words of the sacred, they are also mediums through which response to the sacred can be made. Furthermore, a response to the sacred in and through a commitment of the individual in faithful love and obedience to Jesus Christ both reveals and perfects personhood. Self-fulfillment is a consequence of discipleship, and self-perfection is the continuous effort to eradicate whatever in the self hinders it.

Finally, it should be noted that Häring's religious ethic is thoroughly personalistic. It is grounded in response to the Thou of God in and through the Thou of Christ. The ultimate source of moral obligation is a personal Value who addresses persons in their freedom, and not an impersonal value, concept, or law. There is no place in this ethic for a primacy of impersonal principles as objects of obedience or as the terms of moral activity.

At the same time, this religious ethic opposes an individualistic personalism that radically affirms the "I" at the expense of the "thou" and the "we," that subordinates God, other people, and the community to the realization of the self. This for Häring is contrary to what it means to be a person.

Because the person is made in the likeness of God, he or she reflects the essence of the divine community, namely, "reciprocity of love." This for Häring is what it means to be a person (1968a: 14, 18, 19). This relational nature is not fulfilled solely in the God-person fellowship. Divine community both reveals and grounds human beings' communitarian nature.

> Religion as community with God is also the foundation of the human community, the genuine fellowship of persons. . . . Fellowship with God in word and love develops and fulfills our individual personality (the image of God in us) and at the same time reveals our essentially social nature. Therefore religious living, if it develops its own sound dynamic, places us necessarily in the human community — the word-love fellowship with our fellow men. (1961: 37-38)

What religion discloses about the relational nature of the person, discipleship supports and specifies. Häring sees the person and life of Christ as the clearest expression and example of authentic personalism. Christ's life is lived in absolute openness and self-giving to God and to other people; his death is the final complete self-emptying. Discipleship is in part to struggle against the tendencies toward a self-centered personalism.

Häring's personalism has two important consequences for his moral theology. First, the person has primacy over all that is impersonal, and all that is impersonal (including moral laws) must be in the service of the person. Moral principles and norms are mediations of love and are therefore secondary. Such an orientation not only gives a different weight to moral norms, it also provides a more holistic and person-centered context for evaluating behavior. Second, Häring's great appreciation for persons involves the constant concern that they be recognized, appreciated, and affirmed in their concrete individuality — an emphasis underscored by the biblical influences on Häring's moral theology.

How is it biblically informed? Unlike the moral theology of the manuals, which generally employed scripture to corroborate philosophical arguments, Häring's ethics is permeated by the scriptures, establishing a framework for interpreting all of reality. "Gaining the right vision" is one of Häring's principal concerns. In fact, he considers it a basic task and purpose of moral theology. The "vision" he develops from biblical materials shapes his ethics — its underlying anthropology, its focus on character, its norms and criteria, and its process of moral deliberation. The scriptures are *the* determinative influence for Häring, but they are not the sole influence. He also draws on human experience and the insights of philosophy and the sciences.

Old Testament Perspectives

Häring focuses on two themes in the Hebrew scriptures that are central to their meaning as well as to the present life of the religious person — word and response (1963a: xxii-xxiii; 1978: 471-75). The transcendent God, revealed in gratuitous self-disclosure and issuing an invitation to fellowship (word), evokes certain attitudes and dispositions (response) on the part of the religious individual, namely, grateful praise and faithful obedience. These realities are perhaps best expressed in the biblical notion of covenant. Word and response form the basic structure and dynamic of Häring's religious ethic; they appear in his medical ethics in his discussion of stewardship and in his frequent references to the meaning, vocation, and destiny of the person.

New Testament Perspectives

Christocentrism. Häring's moral theology, as noted earlier, is unmistakably Christocentric; that is, the person of Christ is its basis and core. He writes: "the principle, the norm, the center, and the goal of Christian Moral Theology is Christ. The Law of the Christian is Christ Himself in Person" (1961: vii). In his person and life, Christ is both the revelation of God's self and God's call to fellowship as well as the human acceptance of that invitation in faithful love and obedience. Because of this, he establishes a new relationship between God and people. Christ then embodies and exemplifies the unity of love of God and love of neighbor, and his call to discipleship is an invitation to join in his response to God and to human others. While covenant in the Hebrew scriptures and Christ in the Christian scriptures are the basis of Häring's ethic, it is his understanding of discipleship, or "being-in-Christ," that provides much of its content. Here Häring draws upon Pauline theology, particularly from that in Galatians and Romans. The Pauline concepts of the "freedom of the children of God" (Romans 8:21), the "law of the Spirit" (Romans 8:2), and the "law of Christ" (Galatians 6:2; Romans 2:14) form much of the core of Häring's moral theology. "Christian freedom," especially, permeates all of Häring's work.

Christian freedom. In Pauline theology, freedom is received as a gratuitous gift of God as a consequence of the believer's new existence in Christ. "Being in Christ" requires a new center of loyalty. It does not allow for self-centeredness and self-seeking but rather requires total surrender of the self to God in and through identification with Christ. Only then do believers enjoy the "freedom of the children of God." This is not a freedom to do what one wills but is essentially the freedom to love as exemplified in the person and life of Christ.

By discipleship the believer is freed from the Jewish law and is under the new law of Christ (Romans 8:2; 6:14; 1 Corinthians 9:20; Galatians 6:2; 5:18). That is, as Häring explains, the believer is no longer primarily subject to external, impersonal, minimal laws but rather is subject to the requirements of a faithful, loving, personal relationship (1967a: 19-23). The new law is interior, not imposed from without as was the "old [Mosaic] law" or any other laws. Furthermore, it is not one of requirements, restrictions, and prohibitions, but of ever increasing realization of the "works of the Spirit" (Galatians 5:22-23), the ideals of the Sermon on the Mount (Matthew 5), and the goal of perfect love. Prohibitive commandments (for example, the Decalogue) point to the minimum requirements of love, guidance for Christians still on the way to a more perfect and faithful love, and protections of the common good (1967a: 31, 32). But they are not sufficient for the Christian.

The requirements of love can be discovered by looking to Christ, whom Häring refers to as the "countenance of love" (1971: 126). The true nature of love is revealed in his personality, words, and life. Häring also looks to the Sermon on the Mount for the meaning of love (1971: 128; 1967b: 375-85). Its value lies not in specifying the rightness or wrongness of particular actions but in providing fundamental orientations, attitudes, and motives for action. The Beatitudes are what Häring calls "goal commandments" because they delineate the character of love and point in the direction of greater perfection in one's relationships.

217

Implied here is the need for continuous *conversion* and growth in faithful love in the God-human relationship. Conversion is a central element in Häring's Christian ethics. Drawing particularly from Matthew (4:17; 3:2) and Mark (1:5), Häring interprets conversion to be primarily a transformation of the heart, of one's fundamental way of relating to God and neighbor, and secondarily of one's dispositions, attitudes, motives, and actions, bringing all into ever increasing harmony with existence in Christ. Conversion for Häring does not stop with the individual but extends to a continuing transformation of social and institutional value and belief systems in the direction of fuller embodiments of genuine human values.

An Ethic of Dispositions

Catholic moral theology and secular philosophical ethics have been preoccupied with judgments about the morality of particular actions. This focus has typified most areas of moral inquiry, including the biomedical. In much of his work, Häring has attempted to overcome this tendency and to restore a neglected dimension to moral theology, namely, the centrality of the moral self who performs actions. His concern with the self is not primarily in terms of self-realization but rather with an ever fuller embodiment of "being-in-Christ" in the person's entire character.

"Being-in-Christ," or discipleship, first takes place in the heart of the person, the innermost depths of the self; there she makes the fundamental choice to respond lovingly or unlovingly to the call to fellowship with the sacred as well as to human beings. It is through this basic choice at this affective center that the person determines the moral worth of her self and life and thus the quality of her relationships to self, others, the Absolute Other, and all of created reality. Häring calls this basic choice a person's fundamental option (1978: 87-89, 164-218; 1961: 228-33).

A person's fundamental option affects her knowing and willing. When a decision is made for the good in the depths of the self, a new way of knowing the good and knowing God results. The fundamental option affects the "fundamental attitude," that is, an individual's basic inclination to recognize and respond to the dignity and appeal of Value and values in a characteristic, persistent way. Both contribute to an "instinct of the heart," an innate ("connatural") grasp of what is good

218

and a choice of that good. The fundamental option and attitude need to permeate the entire personality so that they come to be expressed in particular dispositions ("spontaneous impulses" of the heart, persistent over time, in response to particular values) and motives, which in turn influence action (1961: 199-233, 309-10; 1978: 164-218).

Given Häring's ethic of the heart and of dispositions, it is not surprising that he insists more on a commitment of the heart than on specific principles. The more a fundamental option and attitude permeate an individual character, the more he will instinctively choose and do good, and the less he will need external prescriptions and proscriptions. It follows from this also that Häring's mode of moral judgment is more one of "discernment" than of reasoned argument.

This is not an exhaustive discussion of Häring's fundamental moral theology, but it at least provides elements crucial to an understanding of his medical ethics. In brief, Häring's ethics is religious in structure (word-response), biblically and theologically influenced in conception and content (an ethics of discipleship and of Christian freedom), person-centered rather than principle-centered, and more concerned with good character than with right action. Each of these characteristics distinguishes his ethics from traditional Roman Catholic moral theology. With all of this in view, it is now possible to consider Häring's medical ethics.

Toward a Theological Medical Ethics

The Scope of Bioethics and the Task of the Ethicist

David Kelly contends in *The Emergence of Roman Catholic Ethics in North America* that Catholic medical ethics was defined by its practitioners as "the moral theological-philosophical investigation of medical practice" (1979: 221). Its overall objective was to "apply moral principles to the daily professional activity of medical personnel, in order that they, as well as the clergy and laity who might be concerned as moral guide, chaplain, or patient, would know and carry out correct moral procedure" (Kelly 1979: 221). The choice of issues for ethical evaluation was determined on the basis of the everyday needs and practice of medical personnel.

Kelly argues that a shift has occurred in recent medical ethics in terms of the self-definition of the discipline and, consequently, in the type and range of issues considered. "In contrast to this individual approach, today's medical ethics has extended its topical array to include the entire sphere of individual and social, microethical and macroethical problems connected directly or indirectly to the areas of medicine and biology" (1979: 407). This shift, to some extent, is reflected in the more commonly used terms *bioethics* and *biomedical ethics*.

Häring reflects this shift in his *Medical Ethics* (1973). He notes a change in the vision, praxis, and responsibilities of modern medicine brought about largely by advances in biomedical technology. The medical profession, he maintains, no longer finds itself engaged solely in therapeutic medicine but also in preventive medicine, not only concerned about the health of particular organs and individuals but also about the health of individual nations and of the global community. There is an awareness of the consequences of new technologies for the whole of society as well as for the effects of the social and physical environment on the health of the individual and the community (1973: xi; 1976b: 87-88). In light of these changes, Häring believes the physician-patient relationship can no longer be thought of individualistically but must also include a "social-collective responsibility" to the whole of human society (1973: 3).

These changes, Häring argues, also necessitate interdisciplinary dialogue to address not only technological questions but philosophical and theological ones as well. Further, the task of addressing these questions belongs to the entire human community and not only to specialists and should not take place within an individualistic framework but rather from the perspective of "social responsibility for the whole of humanity and for the world environment" (1973: 5).

Häring's broader interests are even more evident in *Ethics of Manipulation* (1976b). Here, he definitely sees the issues as affecting all of humankind, present and future, and his audience is not only the medical practitioner and the patient but the entire human community. "The problems approached here concern not only moralists, members of the medical profession and scientists. They concern all people committed to education in the Church and in the secular world, all legislators, and all mature persons who want to participate in the process of making decisions and arousing consciences about these fundamental questions" (1976b: xii). The repercussions of advances in biology, medicine, and psychology can be a blessing as well as a curse, and so should be the concern of all (1976b: 1-2, 209, 210).

With this change in the nature and scope of bioethics comes an altered perception of the role of the medical ethicist. In traditional Catholic medical ethics, the ethicist tended to be seen as a dispenser of indisputable and once-and-for-all answers arrived at in relative isolation from and exclusion of those directly affected. Instead, Häring describes the ethicist as one who brings moral and religious sensibilities to a broad-based discussion seeking ethical insights and judgments in cooperation with others. The ethicist should be one who listens well, is open to new knowledge and the insights of others, promotes dialogue as an equal partner, suggests avenues to discernment, and offers tentative and limited but important perspectives with regard to the fundamental question: What is the human person and the human vocation? The moral theologian employed in this capacity cannot ignore the research, knowledge, expertise, and experience of the medical and scientific communities.

Häring's work in bioethics should reflect this conception of the nature and scope of medical ethics and of the task of the bioethicist, and to a considerable degree it does. In fact the basic thrust of his medical ethics lies precisely in his attempt to offer morally and religiously informed perspectives about the nature of the human person and human existence as a framework for considering various aspects of health care and the full range of medical technologies. In both *Medical Ethics* (1973) and *Ethics of Manipulation* (1976b), Häring affirms that the primary contribution of theology and of the moral theologian is to promote an "integral vision" of the person, a vision of wholeness and ultimate meaning as a safeguard against all reductionist interpretations (1973: 11, 16-22, 35-38; 1976b: 17, 44, 49-50). He tries to promote this vision by addressing four questions he believes to be pivotal to medical ethics: (1) What is the nature of the human person? (2) What is the meaning of bodily life? (3) What is the meaning of human death? (4) What is the meaning of health and illness? These foundational questions occupy far more of Häring's attention than does his analysis of particular technologies and procedures, and his discussion of them can be said to constitute a good deal of the substance of his medical ethics. In the way he addresses them, one sees the imprint of his fundamental moral theology.

An Integral Vision of the Human

The Nature of the Person

Häring's point of departure for his ethical reflection is the individual. He observes that "the knowledge of man is the basic presupposition of all moral discourse. It is on the great question of 'What is man?' that the moral theologian joins in dialogue with the behavioral sciences and medicine" (1973: 6). He reiterates this in his later work with somewhat greater emphasis on human freedom than in his earlier work. "The final concern and criterion in discussing manipulation is human freedom" (1976a: 50).

At first glance, this might appear to be in contradiction to his religious ethic and to his opposition to an ethics of self-realization. But Häring's understanding of the human, as discussed earlier, includes as an essential element relationship with and responsibility to the divine. The human person is always related to God, who is each person's origin and ultimate destiny (1973: 11, 21, 50). Also, the person's dignity is derived from being made in the image and likeness of God. To respond to the dignity of the person is essentially to respond to value rooted in the divine as well as to a divine presence in this value. This is the structure and dynamic of Häring's religious ethic. As noted previously, Häring believes that the person *is* the appropriate focus of morality, though not its origin and goal.

What for Häring does a theologically grounded holistic vision of the person encompass? First, the body is intrinsic to an adequate understanding of human beings. It is the person's way of being in the world and of having access to the world. The body makes possible the carrying out of the human vocation — worship of God and the love and service of neighbor. It enables being "present and accessible to our fellow man, informed about his needs, able to communicate with him and respond to him" (1971: 49; 1966: 187, 191). This attitude toward the body is based on existentialist and phenomenological thought, and on the Christian doctrines of incarnation and redemption as well. That the Word of God took on a live human body is for Häring the "strongest possible expression of the sum and substance of bodily existence" (1973: 50). Therefore, any disparagement or degradation of the material aspect of human nature would stand in radical opposition to basic Christian beliefs. For both theological and philosophical reasons, Häring firmly rejects any "spiritualistic" anthropology.

At the same time, there is the danger of an overemphasis on bodily aspects of human being, particularly in the practice of medicine. The individual may be reduced to a collection of cells and organs and their functions. He or she may be intentionally or unintentionally viewed as a diseased organ or system of organs instead of these being viewed as part of a larger integrated reality. A biological reductionism, therefore, also does violence to the nature of the person.

What Häring insists upon is viewing the person as an irreducible unity of which materiality (body) and immateriality (spirit) are aspects and not parts. They interpenetrate, are mutually dependent, and, to a great extent, work in conjunction. In short, the person is to be understood as "embodied spirit." It is, however, the spiritual activity of the person that is ultimately of greatest significance because it is this which is most distinguishing of human beings.

Second, though Häring affirms the importance of the body, he rejects the notion that the biological dimension of the person has normative significance, that is, that it determines what is moral and immoral. His approach differs substantially from the approach to natural law typical of traditional Catholic moral theology, which maintains that biological processes, particularly those relating to sex and procreation, are expressive of the will of God. Hence their integrity can never be compromised. It is for this reason that artificial contraception, sterilization, artificial insemination, in vitro fertilization, and the like are condemned by the official Church. Häring acknowledges that a person's biological nature often has "an indicative character," that is, it indicates what usually serves the good of the total person, but this is not always the case (1973: 56). When there is a conflict between preserving biological integrity and the good of the person holistically considered, the latter takes priority. Häring refers to this position as a "desacralization of the biological."[4]

His unequivocal opposition to any sacralization of the physiologi-

---

4. It should be noted here that Häring's "desacralization" also applies to his understanding of human nature. He rejects interpretations of the human that lack a historical element. Human nature, he believes, is developmental, and, because of this, knowledge of it is never exhaustive or unchanging. Such knowledge is, for the most part, empirically and experientially based and is partly gained through an ongoing dialogue between the various sciences and the insights of faith. Häring's treatment of this can be found in "Dynamism and Continuity in a Personalistic Approach to Natural Law" (1968b) and *Morality Is for Persons* (1971: 149-54).

223

cal aspect of human nature flows directly from his personalist anthropology. He situates the meaning of the physiological in the broader
context of human dignity and the totality of the person's relationships.
The biological is in the service of the personal. Preserving the integrity
of the organism can never be to the detriment of "overall well-being
and dignity" (1973: 56). The question for Häring is not whether biomedical technologies respect biological processes but whether they promote the "best possible human health in view of man's total vocation"
(1973: 56). One of the clearest examples of the implications of this
perspective is Häring's handling of artificial contraception and sterilization, both of which he justifies under certain circumstances. With
regard to sterilization, for example, he writes: "Whenever the direct
preoccupation is responsible care for the health of persons or for saving
a marriage (which also affects the total health of all persons involved),
sterilization can then receive its justification from valid medical reasons"
(1973: 90).[5]

Third, Häring's desacralization of the biological is complemented
by what he calls a "resacralization of the person." The person is central
in Häring's medical ethics because he or she is created in God's image
and is a center of consciousness, freedom, and love. These in turn
imply the transcendent origin and destiny of the person, the transcendent source of the person's value and dignity, the relational nature of
human beings, and their cocreativity with God. It also suggests the
nature of the human vocation — which Häring defined in his fundamental moral theology: adoration of God; love, respect, and service to
fellow humans; and a development of the earth to fulfill its own
potentials and to provide a better environment for human flourishing
(1976b: 56; 1973: xi-xii).

A fourth and central component of Häring's theological interpretation of human nature is human stewardship for creation. Because
human beings are created in the image and likeness of God, they have
full stewardship over the earth and are called to be cocreators with the
Creator (1973: 50). This belief arises out of a theology of creation,
incarnation, and redemption: "Belief in *One God, Creator of all things,*

---

5. Häring discusses the morality of contraception and sterilization in several
places: "The Encyclical Crisis" (1969a); "The Inseparability of the Unitive-Procreative
Functions of the Marital Act" (1969b); *Medical Ethics* (1973: 85-89, 90-91); *Ethics of
Manipulation* (1976b: 92-96); *Free and Faithful in Christ* (1981:12-21).

is a call to co-responsibility. . . . By reason of the creation of all things in God and redemption in Jesus Christ, the Christian, more than any other . . . , is entrusted with the task of cultivating the earth and refining his own nature" (1973: 11, 12). For Häring, human interventions in nature are not only permissible but mandatory. He does not consider them an expression of pride but an exercise of God-given freedom and creativity. The unfinished creation, including human biological and psychological nature, is given to humankind not solely for care but also for development (1973: 63; 1976a: 70).

The latter is an important point. Häring believes that the incomplete and developmental character of all created reality, including the human, invites and requires the active intervention of human beings to bring it to fuller realization. No aspect of nature is sacred in the sense of being unalterable and beyond every modifying biomedical intervention. "Creation," he writes, "is an unfinished work that calls for man's cooperation to bring it to greater perfection. And man himself is an unfinished work, called to become an even better image of God" (1976b: 64).[6] The obvious and difficult questions here are, What constitutes the betterment of human and physical nature? How can this be known? and, What criteria can provide guidance? Häring is not as helpful as he might be here, though some aspects of the biblical meaning of stewardship and of his theological anthropology suggest attitudes that circumscribe human creativity.

Creativity for Häring is always cocreativity, the exercise of human ingenuity in cooperation with the Creator and the Creator's purposes. Human beings are "given mastery over what we call 'nature'; but this mastery must never be exercised in a loveless attitude, in a spirit of exploitation, but with reverence for all creation as a word of the one God and Father, as a gift entrusted to us for the benefit of all humankind" (1976b: 68). Responsibility to God and to the human community past and present means that human interventions in nature

---

6. Häring's attitude toward the scope of stewardship, particularly as it relates to human beings, is well illustrated in his treatment of genetics in *Ethics of Manipulation* (1976b: 159-92), especially in his discussion of gene therapy and genetic engineering. Quite typical of his approach is this statement: "On principle, we cannot simply condemn man's desire to improve directly, and even by constructive manipulation of the genes, the genetic basis of human existence. Since man's biological nature is entrusted to his freedom and wisdom, he is, by his very historical nature, the steward of his genetic heritage" (1976b: 183).

ought never be an autonomous and indiscriminate or arbitrary use of power. Furthermore, if creation, as Häring believes, is "word of God," it is, in a sense, sacred. This sacredness engenders an attitude of reverence, respect, and nonexploitation.

Häring's handling of the extent and the manner of human interventions into nature is consistent with his ethics of character. Here as in so many other instances, Häring calls for an inner transformation of the moral agent that will give rise to certain dispositions that in turn will lead to appropriate conduct. The difficulty is in making the move from dispositions to concrete behavior, and in providing guidance for the large numbers whose dispositions have not been transformed in the direction of reverence, cocreativity, and responsibility.

Despite these difficulties, Häring's ethic of stewardship offers a positive, balanced, personalistic, and religious interpretation of the human relationship to nature allowing for the exercise of human freedom, creativity, and ingenuity for the betterment of human beings and of all creation.[7]

The Meaning of Bodily Life

Häring's conception of the meaning of bodily existence is unmistakably informed by the Hebrew and Christian scriptures and is very much consistent with his understanding of the nature and vocation of the person. Bodily existence is a gift of God over which human beings are stewards and is meant to be a time of opportunity (Ephesians 5:16) "for growth in the love of God and neighbor," a time "either to prepare for an everlasting harvest in the community of the saints or for final dissolution in the solidarity of sin" (1976b: 66, 67; 1981: 4). In the language of Häring's general moral theology, it is the time for working out one's fundamental option. Hence, the short period of bodily life is of decisive importance.

Given this, it is precisely the quality rather than the quantity of existence that Häring considers primary, that is, the degree to which the

7. Häring tends to have a positive view of reality, though he does temper it with a realistic notion of sin. He attempts to avoid two extremes: a pessimism that stresses the power of sin and leads to fatalism about the human situation and suspicion and rejection of advances in technology; and an optimism that equates progress in technology with progress in being human. For further discussion, see *Ethics of Manipulation* (1976b: 60-62).

individual is faithful to the human vocation: to grow in relationships, to serve other people and the community of persons, and to enhance the natural world. In fact, efforts at prolonging physical life might well distract from life's true meaning (Matthew 8:35; Luke 9:34; 17:32; John 12:25). With a keen sense of the radical contingency and precariousness of human existence, Häring is emphatic about being vigilant in order to seize the *kairos,* the time that is given, the time of opportunity.[8]

While he emphasizes the gift character of human life and human beings' stewardship of it, "subject to the sovereignty of God," Häring maintains that physical life is not the highest value. "The Gospel is explicit in stating that physical life is not the supreme good; it attains its truth and authenticity to the extent that it serves our neighbor and thus praises God, the giver of life" (1973: 68). Christ typifies the extent to which an individual can dispose of his or her life: "He can even lay it down, if need be, in the service of fellowmen as a witness to faith, hope, and love. In placing his earthly life at the service of brotherhood, man gives the most authentic testimony that he appreciates life as a gift of God" (1973: 69). On the other hand, life is of value even though it may not be productive. Its value rests not on the usefulness but on the dignity of each person.

The Meaning of Human Death

Häring's theological interpretation of death, which prefaces his treatment of moral issues at the end of life, is rather sketchy (1973: 121-27; 1979: 76-81). Two major themes emerge, however. One is directly related to the human vocation, to the meaning of human existence. Death terminates an individual's earthly pilgrimage and thereby finalizes the person's fundamental option. It is a "final momentous decision," which brings either redemption or condemnation. The latter, theological death, is the state of complete alienation of self from relationships, particularly relationship with God. Death can be either the "final event of alienation" or "the moment of consummate unity with Christ and trust in God" (1973: 122; see also 120-25).

---

8. *Kairos* is an important theme in Häring's moral theology. For his most extensive discussion of this concept, see *The Christian Existentialist* (1968a: 70-96) and *Morality Is for Persons* (1971: 104-14).

The second major theme is victory over death through union with Christ.

> Not only was Christ delivered from the grave but all who, through him, open themselves trustingly to his saving solidarity will be delivered from that death which marks participation in the collective alienation of egotists. For them life will never be absurd, nor will death be a catastrophic ending to a meaningless life; for the saving event of Christ's life-death-resurrection transforms death into life's greatest opportunity. Instead of a futile and despairing disfunction with life, it becomes the incomparable breakthrough to life everlasting. (1973: 123)

Central in this perspective is the hope and faith in the fullness of personal life beyond death. It is a "new vision of death," grounded in the sufferings and death of Christ, who overcame its apparent meaninglessness and transformed it into a salvific event.

Häring does not proceed to spell out in any great detail the implications of this Christian interpretation of death. What it can provide in the care of the dying, however, is a structure of meaning and a holistic perspective that transcends a preoccupation with the biological. What is of greater importance for Häring than the cessation of functioning of a biological organism is the meaning of this event in the total existence of the person. This dimension above all needs to be attended to, taking precedence over technical decisions about prolonging life, treatment, and the like. Häring, in fact, believes that it is the physician's responsibility to "transcend his role as servant of biological life," "to share his convictions in relation to a holistic understanding of human existence," and to "search with his patient for the whole impact of death" (1973: 120). Häring's interpretation of human death is an elaboration of his holistic vision of the person, a vision that also influences his understanding of health.

The Meaning of Health and Illness

Häring considers any concept of health that is limited to a concern for the body and bodily functioning inadequate. While acknowledging the importance of physical and physiological well-being and vitality, he maintains that

health cannot be defined from a mere study of the body; we must consider the whole person in his human vocation and final destiny. A comprehensive understanding of human health includes the greatest possible harmony of all man's forces and energies, the greatest possible spiritualization of man's bodily aspect and the finest embodiment of the spiritual. True health is revealed in the self-actualization of the person who has attained that freedom which marshals all available energies for the fulfillment of his total vocation. (1973: 154; see also 1979: 42-48)

While Häring appreciates the interdependence of psychological and spiritual health with biological health, this interdependence cannot obscure the fact that the health of one does not guarantee the health of the other, and that primacy must always be given to the psychological and spiritual dimensions of the individual:

A bubbling bodily vitality which oppresses the spirit comes closer to sickness than does a relatively feeble body, compliant to the spirit and truly subservient to that freedom which is the principal condition and precious fruit of a growing love of God and of one's neighbor. Such a ranking of values does not suggest contempt for human vitality or disdain of bodily strength and robustness; it does not preclude joyousness flowing from bodily well-being. What is disavowed is the making absolute of sheer physical vitality, since this is not a holistically human vitality but one inferior to it. The robust, well-trained and energetic body, toughened and supple, which is an expression and instrument of the spirit and a manifestation of freedom, has a high value. (1973: 154-55)

Häring's final criterion for health would seem to be those conditions that are optimal for the fulfillment of the human vocation. And this need not include physical health.

In fact, Häring does not consider the lack of physical health to be necessarily an entirely negative experience. Illness has redemptive possibilities (1973: 163-67). It can refocus attention on the "imperishable life" and inspire reflection on the meaning of human existence. It may point to personal sin of which a particular disease is a consequence and manifestation, or to the sin of one's ancestors. Or it may uncover a previously hidden egocentrism or lead to experience of human solidarity resulting from reliance on others or even contribute to an attitude of compassion toward others. Illness may be an opportunity for conversion and growth in freedom.

The most tragic element in illness and suffering, for Häring, is the failure to seek out its potential meaning:

> The decisive factor lies in the sick person's sincere quest for the personal message in his illness and for the real possibilities offered and suggested by it for the reorientation of his life. . . .
>
> Illness *per se* has to be seen primarily as a disorder, a chaotic interference with creation; but in that freedom which arises from faith in redemption, the patient and his doctor can fight this chaos and transform the seemingly meaningless into a creative and redeeming event. Illness then becomes an appeal to silence the self-centered ego and to enter more fully into the realm of the freedom of God's children who, *in faith,* place their total trust in him precisely at the moment when their difficulties offer no possibility of self-trust. The true Christian will finally try to see adversity in the light of the pascal mystery. Suffering thus accepted gives a new dimension to life and announces the approach of life everlasting. (1973: 163, 164-65)

Häring cautions, however, that illness not be seen exclusively from the viewpoint of a "mystique of suffering." Healing was an essential part of the mission of Jesus, as was his acceptance of his own suffering and death. The attitude of the Christian, patterned after the example of Christ, might well be the search to heal what can be healed and the acceptance of what cannot (1973: 166). Häring encourages this holistic vision as the perspective of both the patient and the physician.

Normative Criteria and Decision Making

Although Häring's primary concern in working out both a fundamental moral theology and a medical ethics is with the character of the moral agent, he gives some attention to conduct and to specific actions. As might be expected, his approach to this area of moral life is not typical. Interestingly, Häring nowhere seems to address the process of moral deliberation in the sense of what needs to be taken into account in arriving at a moral judgment. Nor does he offer a set of clearly defined moral principles such as one would find in Catholic medical moral textbooks and in the standard philosophical texts in medical ethics. He refers to their importance and necessity, but himself formulates few and rarely employs those explicitly in his own working out of moral problems. Rather, what one finds are theological and anthropological orientations, perspectives, dispositions, and values that he believes are normative. He sometimes refers to them as "objective criteria." And in place of an analytic, systematic, decision-making process, Häring proposes a process of "discernment."[9]

His clearest and most developed statements on this way of arriving at moral judgments are in *Ethics of Manipulation* (1976b). At the beginning of his chapter on "criteria" in that volume, Häring asserts that, before "criteria for judgment," what is needed is the "virtue of critical discernment," which "allows us to distinguish . . . the boundary between the manipulation of things and of biological 'nature' and the manipulation of the human person in his inner sanctuary of freedom" (1976b: 44). This is achieved through people who "excel in wisdom and goodness," that is, the converted. But the objective criteria are also needed in the process of dialogue to resolve the problems of biomedicine. In fact, Häring seems to believe that it is through interdisciplinary dialogue that it is possible to arrive at adequate "criteria for discernment" (1976b: 46).

Häring is even more explicit about discernment as the mode of decision making at the conclusion of this chapter:

> When we speak about objective criteria, we must not allow ourselves those dangerous objectifications that forget the first and basic importance of the persons involved. Objective criteria serve no purpose unless they are freely interiorized by those who have to distinguish between acceptable and unacceptable manipulations. The ethicist has not fulfilled his role if he is aiming only at objective criteria. Our main purpose is to help people to acquire the virtue of critical discernment. . . .
>
> Those whose fundamental option is for freedom and respect for

9. Because of space limitations, I have not dealt with Häring's ethical theory here, but it should be included in a discussion of moral deliberation. Häring affirms the necessity of considering both deontological and teleological factors and of maintaining a harmonious relation between the two. He sees his own methodology as an "option for special emphasis on teleology without, however, excluding all kinds of deontology" (1978: 383). Deontology for Häring is the determination of the characteristics of love. See *Free and Faithful in Christ* (1978: 340-43) and *Ethics of Manipulation* (1976b: 72-78).

all people attain a *connatural sense of the good* that helps them to interiorize the objective criteria. Their *connaturality with the scale of values makes the right choices easy for them.* (1976b: 82, emphasis added)

To develop this virtue of critical discernment, Häring insists on education toward a "morality of responsibility" that includes the imparting of values along with radical conversion.

For Häring, then, the process of arriving at moral judgments regarding biomedical technologies is not primarily one of applying principles to particular procedures. Instead, it consists of a discerning process that involves a converted moral person drawing on his or her experience, the relevant sciences, the views of the other people involved, and the gospel message to determine whether the technologies in question are consistent with and supportive of the meaning and vocation of the human person. The normative input consists in the biblical love command and a vision of the person, along with the values, attitudes, and dispositions flowing from both. Also to be included are the prohibitive commandments and the goal commandments, but specific rules and principles seem to function minimally.

Häring's "normative criteria" need to be considered more thoroughly. In *Medical Ethics,* he proposes as his main criterion the "principle of totality," which must be interpreted from a "perspective of wholeness that considers the total vocation of the human person" (1973: 62). In traditional Catholic medical ethics, totality was understood physically — that is, it referred to the totality of the body rather than of the person. Häring's understanding and formulation of totality expresses the substance of his anthropology: *"the dignity and well-being of man as a person in all his essential relationships to God, to his fellowmen and to the world around him"* (1973: 62; see also 63, 64). He employs this principle to assess a whole range of medical procedures and technologies.

Whereas in *Medical Ethics* (1973) the criterion for ethical decision making is built on "human dignity," "wholeness," and the "vocation of man," the emphasis in *Ethics of Manipulation* (1976b) is primarily on freedom and its growth. The shift in language may be due to the different concerns of the two works. In the former, Häring addresses fundamental questions such as the meaning of the person and of life, death, and suffering, considers the proper relationship of doctors and

232

patients, and takes up an ethical evaluation of such things as birth control, sterilization, organ transplants, prolonging life, and psychotherapy. In the latter book, he deals with biomedical technologies that more directly fall under the category of "manipulation." Understood positively, manipulation is the "beneficial planned change of nature . . . , piloting the biological or psychological nature or functions to the advantage of persons and social relationships" (1976b: 5). Negatively, the term refers to a view of the world and of people in which everything is perceived simply as raw material for technical production and consumption. Häring identifies several realms of manipulation, including biomedicine. Within this area, he focuses on various forms of behavior modification, chemical and surgical alterations of the brain, genetic engineering, therapy and counseling, and alternate methods of human reproduction.

Häring sees what he calls the "one dimensional" perspective as the greatest threat emerging from a scientific and technological society. Essentially, it is an anthropological reductionism, an understanding and definition of persons from a limited vision that does not do justice to the fullness of human reality. Persons become confused with things. To counter these various threats, Häring seeks the "ethical boundaries of manipulation." What is required is a "theory of essential human values" (1976b: 45), including wholeness, human sacredness, and freedom.

Häring is as emphatic about a holistic understanding of the person in *Ethics of Manipulation* as he was in *Medical Ethics*. Only when people are viewed holistically will their true nature be understood and appreciated, thereby helping to avoid reductionistic interpretations and the inclination toward unacceptable manipulation. The task of keeping a holistic perspective in view is incumbent upon all. This requires first of all that each attend to all the dimensions of his own self, his own nature and vocation (1976a: 56). In effect, Häring is calling for a conversion of the self as a weapon against reductionism in a technological society, a conversion that involves an authentic understanding and living out of one's human vocation. Any medical treatment or technology "that jeopardizes the vision of human wholeness or the desire to reach out for wholeness is," for Häring, "a road to unacceptable manipulation" (1976a: 56). "Wholeness," then, in *Ethics of Manipulation,* seems to point to what the principle of totality states more explicitly in *Medical Ethics* (1973: 57).

As important as this concept is for Häring, however, it is freedom that stands out as his fundamental normative emphasis: "The final

233

concern and criterion in discussing manipulation is human freedom" (1976b: 50; see also 57, 71). Häring seems to have two modes of freedom in mind. One is the freedom or the capacity to effect change — the freedom of creative stewardship (1976b: 50-51, 68-72). As such, there are normative requirements in its use. It ought to be employed in a spirit of reverence and gratitude, with the recognition of all the earth as the gift of the Creator.

The other mode of freedom is at once more basic and more important. It is the freedom to be true to one's identity as a personal being. Häring expresses this as "transforming human life in the direction of wholeness and fulfillment" (1976b: 51). The exercise of freedom (creativity) in the personal world means respecting and fostering what human beings are meant to be and become. For Häring, the highest expression of creative freedom is enabling and promoting relationships with God and with neighbor, in effect fulfilling one's nature, vocation, and the meaning of one's existence, and helping others to achieve the same (1976b: 51; see also 50, 57, 61).

As one might expect, Häring points to Christ as the model for all of the meaning of freedom for love and service, of "openhearted relationships," and of mutual respect and love. In addition, the Beatitudes point to characteristics of true freedom and respect for human persons and to the proper attitudes toward the gratuitousness of God's creation — adoration, thanksgiving, and generosity (1976b: 79).

Some uses of freedom — for self-affirmation and self-exaltation, for getting power over others and manipulating them in the service of the self — contribute to alienation from self, others, and God. Such negative uses of freedom objectify human beings. And, as Häring maintains, before another person one should "stand in awe and reverence, in respect for each person's freedom" (1976b: 53). This is Häring's criterion of *respect for human dignity*. The task of ethical reflection is to discern which technologies threaten or violate this dignity. "If we are to esteem ourselves as human persons," says Häring, "we have to oppose any action that endangers or practically denies anyone's humanity, his unique dignity and capacity to grow in freedom" (1976b: 55).

Hence, freedom and dignity are intimately related to Häring's basic theological anthropology (person-in-relation) and, in effect, are simply another way of approaching and expressing it. Perhaps it would be more accurate to say that freedom is the *condition* that makes possible realization of one's nature as person-in-relation and that dignity flows from that nature. Totality is Häring's concise statement of essential human nature, dignity points to its intrinsic value, and freedom is the capacity to achieve it.

Such are Häring's normative considerations and his approach to moral deliberation, and there is much here to commend. His focus on persons holistically considered and their relationships, in conjunction with his sensitivity to individual uniqueness and context (which have not been discussed here), can contribute to a better grasp of situations that may in turn lead to a more "fitting" moral response. Too quick a reference to general principles can lead to a superficial understanding of what is going on. His appeal to discernment not only introduces an affective dimension to moral deliberation but also involves the moral agent at a deeper level of the self and places far more responsibility on the agent's own moral development.

This appeal to discernment, on the other hand, is the source of a possible inadequacy in Häring's understanding of moral deliberation. It seems to assume a converted moral subject — someone who is relatively clear about his or her nature, vocation, and destiny and whose life is faithful to them. But when the moral subject is not converted (which is probably more often the case), there is greater chance for error in the intuitive discernment of proper values and behavior. Clear principles and norms, together with a more reasoned approach to making moral judgments, might be not only a helpful supplement but a much-needed one.

Conclusion

Reflecting on the role of religion in bioethics, Courtney Campbell has observed that "the nature and purpose of life, and the place of health, medicine, suffering, and death within a vision of human nature and destiny, while integral to religious discourse, are common human questions of meaning that often seem peripheral in the quandary-centered concerns of bioethics." In light of this, a major contribution of the religious traditions to the field of bioethics might well be "to broaden our moral vision by raising issues of existential interest that are not typically addressed in contemporary bioethics" (Campbell 1991: 8). Campbell's comment aptly describes Bernard Häring's importance for bioethics. In contrast to traditional Roman Catholic medical ethics (and even some of the work being done by revisionist moral theologians)

ON BERNARD HÄRING

and the commonly accepted philosophical approach to medical ethics in the United States, Häring articulates an understanding of fundamental human experiences — bodily existence, death, health, and illness — within the context of a theologically informed vision of the nature, vocation, and destiny of the human person. Whether or not those working in the field of medical ethics happen to agree with the content of Häring's "vision" or are satisfied with its formulation or the adequacy of its development, there is yet something instructive in his project. He has endeavored to bring the convictions of his religious tradition to bear upon the interpretation of several fundamental dimensions of human existence that always lie just beneath the surface of the quandaries and too often remain there uncovered and unexamined. The resulting vision of reality and context of meaning provide a far richer approach to medical ethics than those that tend to focus on principles and quandaries and to abstract actions from the persons who perform them and persons from the contexts in which they live and act. Häring's emphasis on an approach to persons considered holistically and in the context of their various relationships is likely to contribute to a fuller understanding of what is going on in the particular situation and to a more fitting response than one that applies principles to cases. In addition, a number of Häring's central ideas suggest potentially fruitful directions of inquiry for dealing with other inadequacies in both theological and philosophical modes of doing medical ethics. His conception of the person as inherently relational and social counterbalances a pervasive individualistic notion; his insistence on responsibility counterbalances a preoccupation with rights; his concern with the quality and development of moral character broadens the scope of moral inquiry beyond concerns about what to do. Perhaps of greatest importance is that he illustrates how medical ethics can be construed theologically and what difference theology can make.

References

Beauchamp, Tom L., and James F. Childress. 1979. *Principles of Biomedical Ethics.* New York: Oxford University Press.
Campbell, Courtney. 1991. "Religion and Moral Meaning in Bioethics." *Hastings Center Report* 20: 4-10.

Curran, Charles E. 1982. "Free and Faithful in Christ: A Critical Evaluation." *Studia Moralia* 20: 145-75.

Gustafson, James M. 1978. "Theology Confronts Technology and the Life Sciences." *Commonweal* 105: 386-92.

Häring, Bernard. 1961. *The Law of Christ, Volume One: General Moral Theology,* trans. E. G. Kaiser. Westminster, Md.: Newman Press.

————. 1963a. *The Law of Christ, Volume Two: Special Moral Theology,* trans. E. G. Kaiser. Westminster, Md.: Newman Press.

————. 1963b. *Le sacré et le bien: religion et moralité dans leurs rapports mutuels,* trans. R. Givord. Paris: Éditions Fleurus.

————. 1966. *The Law of Christ, Volume Three: Special Moral Theology,* trans. E. G. Kaiser. Westminster, Md.: Newman Press.

————. 1967a. *Christian Maturity,* trans. Arlene Swidler. New York: Herder and Herder.

————. 1967b. "The Normative Value of the Sermon on the Mount." *Catholic Biblical Quarterly* 29: 375-85.

————. 1968a. *The Christian Existentialist: The Theology of Self-Fulfillment in Modern Society.* New York: New York University Press.

————. 1968b. "Dynamism and Continuity in a Personalistic Approach to Natural Law." In *Norm and Context in Christian Ethics,* ed. Gene Outka and Paul Ramsey, 199-218. New York: Scribner's Sons.

————. 1969a. "The Encyclical Crisis." In *The Catholic Case for Contraception,* ed. Daniel Callahan, 71-91. Toronto: Macmillan.

————. 1969b. "The Inseparability of the Unitive-Procreative Functions of the Marital Act." In *Contraception: Authority and Dissent,* ed. Charles E. Curran, 176-92. New York: Herder and Herder.

————. 1971. *Morality Is for Persons.* New York: Farrar, Straus and Giroux.

————. 1973. *Medical Ethics.* Notre Dame, Ind.: Fides Publishers.

————. 1976a. *Embattled Witness: Memories of a Time of War.* New York: Seabury Press.

————. 1976b. *Ethics of Manipulation: Issues in Medicine, Behavior Control and Genetics.* New York: Seabury Press.

————. 1978. *Free and Faithful in Christ, Volume One: General Moral Theology.* New York: Seabury Press/Crossroad Publishing.

————. 1979. *Free and Faithful in Christ, Volume Two: The Truth Will Set You Free.* New York: Seabury Press/Crossroad Publishing.

————. 1981. *Free and Faithful in Christ, Volume Three: Light to the World.* New York: Seabury Press/Crossroad Publishing.

Healy, Edwin. 1956. *Medical Ethics.* Chicago: Loyola University Press.

Kass, Leon. 1990. "Practicing Ethics: Where's the Action?" *Hastings Center Report* 20: 5-12.

Kelly, David F. 1979. *The Emergence of Roman Catholic Medical Ethics in North America.* New York: Edwin Mellen Press.

Kelly, Gerald A. 1958. *Medico-Moral Problems.* St. Louis, Mo.: Catholic Hospital Association.

Kenny, John. 1952. *Principles of Medical Ethics.* Westminster, Md.: Newman Press.

McFadden, Charles. [1949] 1961. *Medical Ethics.* 5th ed. Philadelphia: F. A. Davis.

O'Donnell, Thomas. 1956. *Morals in Medicine.* Philadelphia: F. A. Davis.

MEDICAL ETHICS AND THEOLOGY

The Accounting of the Generations

MARTIN E. MARTY

NINE YOUNGER experts who bring theology to bear in the field of medical ethics have written in this volume (in pieces originally published in *Second Opinion*) on the work of nine of their predecessors from the two previous generations. These were mentors who began to be active after mid-century and who have made their mark during the most recent third of this century. (The dividing line between such generations, of course, is never neat, so there is some overlap.) Assuming that these writers have done a reasonably accurate job of condensing, presenting, and criticizing the thought of the modern shapers of their discipline — most of whom drew upon and reworked ancient traditions of moral and religious discourse — we can use their essays as a valuable and revealing body of thought for appraising the enterprise as a whole.

One way to grasp something of this whole is to picture some archaeologists, centuries from now, unearthing this collection. Suppose they found no other traces of such lore as this surviving from our time, no other documents to probe. If they could work only with this sort of Dead Sea Scrolls of theologically informed medical ethics, what would they conclude?

To make the game of appraisal worthwhile, we have to hypothesize that the choice of figures for analysis was representative. It would be impossible, of course, to get complete agreement among everyone about who should be in this canon. The most obvious missing candidate would be the recently deceased Joseph Fletcher, who many would say was the pathbreaker in the 1950s and who lived on to continue his radical love-centered (and eventually post-theological or nontheological, agnostic) probing. Likewise, a footnote in the essay on Immanuel Jakobovits mentions numerous candidates in the second generation of Jewish medical ethicists, peers of some of the Christians in this collection, who might well have been included: for example, J. David Bleich and Moshe Tendler from Orthodoxy, or David Feldman and Seymour Siegel from Conservatism (Gellman 1991: 115). Were there space for more, certainly Charles Curran at least would be a credible Roman Catholic nominee. All such additional choices would have provided important exceptions to some of the generalizations that follow, just as much of their work would complement what these nine writers have analyzed. It is hard to say who *else* might belong, but there is no question that these nine *do*.

The company of these thinkers would provide a clue about vocations to archaeologists of the future: for instance, that theologically informed medical ethics might have been pursued in the rabbinate — no parish priests or ministers happen to be here — but that the conventional abode for such inquiry was the university or the graduate theological school connected with universities.

If the archaeologists were to find a comparable collection from the subsequent and thus current generation, they would find women represented as decisive thinkers. Women were not so active between the 1950s and the 1970s; only one is among the authors of this collection. Why? Legal scholar Dena Davis (1991) has shown why it was difficult for women to master the vastnesses of rabbinic texts without which one could not "do" Jewish medical ethics: they were not in the rabbinate, where acquaintanceship with the documentary tradition and habituation to the ethos of these studies occurred. One generation later, women had joined the rabbinic ranks or had found ways to join the company of lay scholars in universities.

Similarly, archaeologists of the future would have to imagine their way back into our times to understand another distortion in the collection: since Catholicism did not ordain women as priests, American Catholic women, though they had access to the documentary tradition out of which Catholic ethics emerges and also had some precedents, especially in religious orders of times past, had less chance to make their way in the theological academy. Even without their ordination, however, Catholicism in the subsequent generation produced numerous leaders among women who would be candidates for inclusion in a future round.

As for Protestants, where the ordination of women became common during the part of the century under scrutiny, it is hard to remember that at mid-century only two or three women held tenured chairs in notable Protestant theological schools. The development of religious studies in universities and the diffusion of women's presence in all the theological disciplines meant that the period from 1950 to 1970 was the last from which women would have been excluded in a representative collection.

One could point to other scholarly cohorts who had less chance than others to leave their mark: Eastern Orthodox Christianity was only coming to be a sufficient cultural presence in North America. Scholars in African-American Christianity, Islam, or Asian religion rarely branched into medical ethics. What we have, then, is not only a portrait of a company of scholars but a glimpse of the culture in the academy, church, and clinic after the middle of the twentieth century.

The lore and ethos on which these scholars drew came to be denominated, somewhat artificially, as *Judeo-Christian,* and it would be this tradition alone that the diggers in some remote future would uncover. Given the great differences in philosophies of history subscribed to by Jews and Christians, the naming of this tradition appeared to some to have been a political invention designed to suit the situation of American pluralism and also to do justice to a strong Jewish cultural presence.

In Marc Gellman's (1991) tracing on these pages, it would become obvious to the future scholars that Rabbi Immanuel Jakobovits did not draw on Christian sources; neither, in these condensed presentations of their thought, did the Christian eight make any references to the rabbinical tradition. When Americans speak of any common tradition, they are usually talking about the use Christians make of the Hebrew scriptures, which they call the Old Testament. Christians interpret these scriptures in vastly different ways than do the Jews, but their reliance on them is genuine and profound.

In passing, one might note that if Christian readers found the writings of Rabbi Jakobovits to be somewhat remote, arcane, and not easily accessible, so Christian exposition similarly would not check out as the linguistic or conceptual "coin of the realm" to most intellectuals

241

in the generally secular culture of America, whose published works would no doubt be available to tomorrow's archaeologists. At the same time, the discourse of these Christian ethicists would be remote from that of most Christian believers, who were not, for the most part, theologically informed in any technical sense. That is, an archaeologist pondering the pop and folk literature of Christianity in these times would find that the ethicists necessarily drew on specialized language to communicate.

Could the archaeologists in a remote tomorrow rely on these writings, then, as having been addressed to or having issued from the communities of substantial numbers of Americans? The answer has to be an emphatic yes. These future archaeologists may not stumble upon parched opinion polls — though, given the prevalence of polls and the relative scarcity of theological ethics writings, they stand a good chance of coming across some — but they would find that as late as 1990, polls that relied on large or small samples of the citizenry found 85 percent of the population considering themselves to be Christian. Another 3 percent of the public considered themselves to be Jewish. Six out of ten Americans considered themselves Protestant; one out of four, Catholic. The main sources of modern theological ethics are the texts on which the faith communities of a significant majority of Americans were founded.

The probing archaeologists who looked beyond denominational identifications to find the sites of theological work would find that it occurred chiefly in the academy. The newer field of "clinical ethics," in which medical doctors predominated, also developed during this period, but no one who possessed an M.D. and a Ph.D. had yet become a pace-setting writer (as opposed to practitioner) in this field, at least not where theological concerns were present.

The university location was an important element in the scholars' work. Some of them may have been responsible to ecclesiastical bodies, but their credentialing came chiefly from fellow academics — from professors, not from higher clergy. When their work was analyzed, it was by other professors. In the case of some of the Catholics, their church body might monitor or criticize their work, but the academy was free to prize what the current church leadership censored or treated warily. The rules of the game in theological ethics were chiefly set by the academy.

Medical ethics in the decades after mid-century was in the hands

of philosophers and theologians. Other seminary disciplines, like practical theology or clinical pastoral care, underwent considerable development after mid-century, but their articulators did not specialize in
ethics, and they addressed other elements of the human condition. The
concerns in these disciplines often complemented those of the ethicists,
as in the case of the overlapping approaches to themes like suffering.
But differentiation and specialization dictated that the credible voices
in theological ethics undergo technical training developed through a
lifelong familiarity with a particular set of texts and approaches.

If one had asked the nine ethicists "back in the twentieth century"
to write ordinary job descriptions for themselves, how would they read?
It is always a bit startling to think of one- or two-word descriptions;
"Martin Luther, Professor of Old Testament," for example, sounds different from "Martin Luther, Reformer," the latter a title that would not
have been appropriate for *Who's Who in Germany, 1517.*

In the present sequence, Rabbi Jakobovits would be described no
doubt simply as rabbi, the others as professors. Only one or two would
say they were professors of medical ethics. The rest were self-described
as theological ethicists who had something important to say about medical ethics or who sometimes even made it their chief field of application.
But none of them sought "instant relevance" as commentators on the
hard cases they all had to take up. They exercised more durable influence
because they gave most attention to the matrix and context of theology
and ethics as background to the medical ethics world. None would have
chosen the term *bioethicist,* a coinage of the period, as a self-description.

For William F. May, the task of academic theologians was to
"clarify, interpret, and criticize" the abundant religious realities sur-
rounding them (Meilaender 1989: 107). Allen D. Verhey (1988) saw
James M. Gustafson pursuing Christian theology as "an intellectual discipline undertaken within the context of the faith and tradition of the
Christian community, where the experience of an ultimate power is
nurtured and informed by the memory of certain religiously significant
events, concepts, and symbols." Meanwhile, ethics is "an intellectual
discipline that reflects upon a dimension of human experience, . . .
denoted 'moral'" (Verhey 1988: 105). Ron P. Hamel (1991: 116) wrote
of Bernard Häring that this priest saw the ethicist as "one who brings
moral and religious sensibilities to a broad-based discussion seeking
ethical insights and judgments in cooperation with others."

Ethicists in those years did find zones where practice counted in their work. Illustrative were the involvements of Richard McCormick on an array of panels such as those of the American Hospital Association, American Fertility Society, National Hospice Organization, the Ethics Advisory Board of the Department of Health, Education and Welfare, and the President's Commission on Bioethics (Cahill 1988: 109). The citation of the writings of James F. Childress in landmark instances (Campbell 1989: 131) showed that these professors by no means led sequestered lives doing work with high levels of abstraction and remoteness. Anything but that. Still, the university disciplines to which they contributed helped define them and shape their work.

The various essayists treated these nine thinkers as members of a generation and a half. They could not have produced a collection such as this back in 1950. Bernard Häring first published his landmark work *The Law of Christ* in English in 1961 (Hamel 1991: 110). The other senior figure, Rabbi Jakobovits, had produced *Jewish Medical Ethics* in 1959, but Marc Gellman (1991: 97, 115) thinks it inappropriate to speak of the new era in medical ethics before 1967, when the Harvard Medical School advanced new criteria for brain death. The pioneer of Protestantism (in this company), Paul Ramsey, brought focus to his work with *The Patient as Person* in 1970. The timing is important: it was during the 1960s, a period of tumult in churches — the Vatican Council (1962-65) in Catholicism and various versions of "radical" and "secular" theology predominating in Protestantism were highlights — that theological interest in medical ethics grew. This was a time when there were cultural indications that America was turning radically secular, rejecting Jewish and Christian traditions, making it harder than before to apply biblical and ecclesiastical norms to the fields of medicine and well-being.

The cultural situation may have occasioned what almost all the essays suggest: that the ethicists regarded their work as fundamentally problematic. How could they get a hearing for religion, theology, and church in a culture where religion was pervasive, theology vital, and the church strong, but where academic and medical professional elites had no patience for and often showed disdain for all three? Conversely, how could they get religious bodies to overcome their suspicion of so much in medicine, technology, and philosophy, so that their resources could be brought to bear on people who faced illness and sought health? How could they speak the theological word in the medical world?

Given their interpretations of their environment as being uncaring and sometimes hostile, it is a marvel that these theological ethicists persevered and made any mark. At times, some of them wavered and adopted the "ordinary secular" language of philosophical ethics in many settings; one might even say that the isolation of theological motifs in these nine thinkers when appraised for the journal *Second Opinion,* which paid special attention to such motifs, may make them sound more explicitly theological than they tended to be when they spoke up in clinics or universities.

Allen D. Verhey (1988: 104) tells of James M. Gustafson's poise: "He acknowledged that there were sometimes good reasons for silence about theological convictions" in commentaries on medical ethics, but, Verhey went on, Gustafson "more vigorously pointed out good reasons to lament this silence. Chief among these was the simple truth that faithful members of religious communities want to live and die and work and care with faithful integrity, not just with impartial rationality."

American culture of the time, in a term William May once used, "reeked of religion," but it was also secular in many dimensions, and that created problems. So did pluralism, as all these thinkers recognized. Stanley Hauerwas, citing Alasdair MacIntyre's *After Virtue,* made that particularly clear. "MacIntyre holds that people today live in a morally fragmented world, that there is no coherent morality" (Lammers 1988: 131). Hauerwas and others asked why, in the midst of all the fragmentation, one mode — the one based on secular rationality alone — should be privileged and have hegemony, if not monopoly.

The society had made one form of discourse apparently easy for itself by conventionally turning religion into "a private affair." Yet religion clearly had public consequences. Patients brought their private meanings into the pluralist setting of the hospital, where they often reasoned about morality in ways that did not match those of the philosophical ethicists, especially whenever they were attentive to religious norms, the ones with which theologians worked. This secular-pluralist concept of the times conditioned and colored everything that this band of theological ethicists analyzed and proposed. Yet, as presented here, they did not gripe or sulk; they set out to do something about the situation. It would be absurd to say that they or anyone else had won their way and become privileged. But as the second half of the century unfolded, the voice of religion and theology was increasingly heard in sectors of the academic and clinical ethics world, thanks in no small measure to thinkers like the 18 (counting both the subjects and the authors) in this collection.

Lest it appear to the archaeologists centuries from now that a hostile world around them simply united this band of theological ethicists, let it be noted that they in various ways also had adopted modes of thinking which their own spiritual and theological ancestors would have called *secular*. While numbers of them stressed that death did not have the last word with human existence, they found talk of *transcendence* more congenial than the language of supernatural *otherworldliness*.

Pluralism is indeed represented among them; there were vast differences not only between Jakobovits and the Christians, or between the three Catholics and the five Protestants, but also among those in each camp: James Childress and Stanley Hauerwas represented opposite poles on most vital positions, including their originating points, the communities they would address, and many of their intentions and goals.

One thing the archaeologists would discover is that these thinkers all *did* have in common a resistance to the trendy "more secular than thou" theology of many radical Jewish and Christian thinkers of their period. Only two or three of them (perhaps Jakobovits, Grisez, and Ramsey) would have been considered conservative by their ecclesiastical colleagues, but they were all traditional in the sense that they engaged in *ressourcement*, a profound revisiting of and drawing upon their traditions, and they were more ready to reinterpret than to reject classic symbols and statements.

This tendency shows up most in their frank and up-front stress on God. Were they Buddhist or Confucian thinkers they might be religious but not theistic, God not being the subject of religious thought or the object of faith in such traditions. Ron Hamel quoted an important positioning statement by James Gustafson in which he criticized religious ethicists working in medical ethics — sometimes including thinkers in this collection — for too frequently abandoning their responsibility to do Christian ethics theologically. "The relation of their moral discourse to any specific theological principles or even to a definable religious outlook is opaque," he complained. Hamel also cited physician-philosopher Leon Kass: "Perhaps for the sake of getting a broader hearing, perhaps not to profane sacred teachings or to preserve a separation between the things of God and the things of Caesar, most religious ethicists entering the public practice of ethics leave their special insights at the door and talk about 'deontological vs. consequentialist,' 'autonomy vs. paternalism,' 'justice vs. utility,' just like everybody else."

246

At least in the presentations here, which focused on the theological dimension, the thinkers made some effort not to be "just like everybody else" (Hamel 1991: 111).

Rabbi Jakobovits, insistent that he should speak only out of Jewish texts to the Jewish community, made no compromises in efforts to write with immediate relevance for the general medical and ethical communities that he professed he intended to reach. The Roman Catholics, on the other hand, had the easiest time showing that their tradition at least *intended* to aspire to the universal, through the time-honored concept of *natural law*. Yet there were open disagreements between a neoscholastic Catholic like Germain Grisez, who relied strongly on a kind of unreconstructed usage, and Richard McCormick, whom Grisez criticized for reinterpreting natural law teaching too much. For Grisez, "a moral philosophy within the natural law tradition sees actions as right insofar as they help to realize the full potential of human nature and wrong insofar as they frustrate the full realization of that potential." But he then fleshed out natural law in such a way that it ruled out all "artificial" birth control. His fellow Catholic Richard McCormick and many other Catholic thinkers of the times did not concur with him, an indication that natural law was itself a divisive issue that settled little and a problematic tie on the part of some religions to secular ethics in American culture (Hanink 1990: 87). On the basis of his version of natural law thinking, Grisez could say with comfort that there were moral absolutes and could spell them out (Hanink 1990: 93), something that other natural law thinkers were less ready to do and that the general ethicists' community dismissed as being confessionally Catholic.

Richard McCormick used Catholic natural law thinking as a bridge to other approaches, but he also wrote that "there are factors at work in moral convictions that are reasonable but not always reducible to the clear and distinct ideas that the term 'human reason' can mistakenly suggest." McCormick also used a frankly hermeneutical approach that Grisez would reject. That is, for him there is no stable meaning to a text; what the interpreter brings to it affects the interpretation. Thus: "the Catholic church *interprets natural law; it does not simply transmit revelation*," and that fact produced problems for Catholic and non-Catholic alike (Cahill 1988: 112). McCormick, on the other hand, drew fire from Hauerwas and his kind for contending that the substance or content of Christian moral thinking was not different from what one could deduce from natural law reasoning. The priest's six main themes were designed to suggest this: "the value of life as a basic but not absolute good; the inclusion of 'nascent' life in the good of human life; the definition of the highest and only absolute good in human life in terms of love of God and neighbor; the essential sociality of persons; the unity of the 'spheres' of life giving and love making; and the normative value of heterosexual, permanent marriage" (Cahill 1988: 116).

Not only Catholics aspired to address the universal situation with a translatable ethic; James Childress among the Protestants leaned furthest toward the "universal" — to some of his critics he looked quite like a secular rationalist with a reminiscent Quaker piety. This did not mean that he was not theologically informed or given to what James M. Gustafson called "natural piety," or even Quaker piety! Explicitly, Childress's Quaker impulse asked him to be preoccupied with "answering that of God in every person," an approach indicating "a universalistic impulse" that required the ethicist "to take account of and be accountable to non-theologically informed positions."

Childress, as an author of medical ethics textbooks, had considerable influence beyond theological circles and became one of the prime keepers of the secular philosophical canon and code. In his outline, medical ethics was devoted simply to *nonmaleficence, beneficence, utility, justice,* and *respect for persons* (sometimes spelled out as *autonomy*). In all cases he connected these themes with divine *agape,* or love. But Childress's critics questioned whether the theological connection was anything but merely an evidence of nostalgia or arbitrariness (Campbell 1989: 121-23).

Hauerwas, as already noted, spoke from the opposite pole, from which vantage Childress's thought would be called liberal. "Liberalism as an approach to morality is flawed because it presupposes a universal morality. For Hauerwas, there were moralities only of particular communities; a universal morality is an illusion," even, Hauerwas insisted, when it came through Catholic natural law reasoning (Lammers 1988: 131). Yet, said Stephen E. Lammers, "Hauerwas thinks that he is advancing a 'natural theology' when he discusses medicine," and did not want to be dismissed as merely confessional or sectarian. He simply saw "no way to speak except within the confines of a particular language, devoted to a peculiar story of a special, e.g., Christian, community" (Lammers 1988: 138).

However much the thinkers might have disagreed with each other on how the talk about God connected with "natural," "universal," or

248

"other" languages and concerns, their own talk about God was open, persistent, and focal. Gustafson would have found few reasons to accuse these colleagues, as here represented, of muting or muffling their witness to God at the grounding of theological ethics, including in its medical applications. For theologians *not* to talk centrally about *theos* might seem oxymoronic, but there was a good deal of oxymoronism running around in the decades when these thinkers made their statements.

One wonders, however, whether it was not precisely the frankness of their God-talk that secular colleagues found impressive even as it raised problems. The theologically informed ethicists who fled for cover, lost nerve, covered up their tracks, or found no ways to focus on God seemed to have less influence than did their expressive co-believers (though Daniel Callahan, who began as a lay Catholic theologian, moved clearly and cleanly out of the orbit of faith and theology and yet had profound influence). The lesson that might be taken from these theo-centered if not necessarily "God-intoxicated" reasoners is that one cannot have it both ways: to establish one's credentials as a theologian and then be embarrassed about one's chief subject.

Rabbi Jakobovits, as presented by Marc Gellman, did not talk so much about God as about the Law given through Moses and expounded by the prophets and rabbis, but there was no question at all about the rabbi's theocentrism. The God to whom such as the rabbi testified and whose bearing they would see in relation to human persons and in ethical discourse is rather consistently the One described by Gustafson as "Creator, Sustainer, Judge, and Redeemer" (Verhey 1988: 106). None of the nine were pragmatists, cocksure elaborators on the ways of God as if they could know this God in exhaustive ways. Yet they were also not agnostic; whether through experience, revelation, apprehension of divine self-disclosure, reckoning with classic texts, being moved by stories, or by reason, they spoke of some measure of knowability directed to the divine.

On these terms, Gustafson issued a "call for piety to form the intention to relate to all things in ways appropriate to their relation to God." This formation, he argued, could happen only when "the transcendent God cannot be altogether unknowable, an empty cipher behind or beyond all human attempts to describe God." So, in Verhey's reticent description of a diffident Gustafson, "the character and purposes of the transcendent God are not unknowable, even if they are not fully and exhaustively knowable. The transcendent God is not a totally unknown God, even if God can be known only by analogy" (Verhey 1988: 111). Readers who a priori ruled out the possibility of intelligible discourse by reference to a symbol of the Other ("God") to which over 90 percent of their fellow citizens somehow related positively would find little point in pursuing the thought of these theological ethicists except as a curiosity.

Eight of the nine thinkers, as already observed, were Christian. "Can medical ethics be Christian?" Gustafson once asked (Verhey 1988: 111), and he answered his question affirmatively, if with many qualifications and complications. Admittedly, when theological ethics turned Christocentric, as it did with Stanley Hauerwas and Bernard Häring, more qualifications and complexifications appeared. Childress spoke of God's activity "expressed theologically as creating, ordering, and redeeming," and linked this with anthropological corollaries in the human situation "being understood as created, fallen, and redeemed" (Campbell 1989: 125). He may have spoken positively of Jesus Christ, but Christ was not integral to his ethics.

Häring, on the other hand, made much of "discipleship" (Hamel 1991: 111) without trying to separate himself from the larger ethical and medical communities. Hamel summarized his accents: "Häring's ethics is religious in structure (word-response), biblically and theologically influenced in conception and content (an ethics of discipleship and of Christian freedom), person-centered rather than principle-centered, and more concerned with good character than with right action." All of these accents separated him from traditional, pre–World War II, pre–Vatican II ethics (Hamel 1991: 115). It was the "Christian freedom" motif, tied to the figure of Jesus Christ, that was least immediately translatable to the larger community.

Hauerwas expressed little interest in anything but the story of Israel and the Christian church, as focused in Jesus Christ. Stephen E. Lammers summarized: "Christians must give primary witness to the person of Jesus, Jesus as he is presented in the Gospels. . . . [Hauerwas recognized] that the Jesus presented [in the scriptural texts] is not the 'historical' Jesus but Jesus as he was understood by those whose lives he had transformed. This . . . is all that we have and all we can know." In Jesus came witness to the kingdom of God — theocentrism therefore triumphed — and to discipleship. The Christian community, Hauerwas argued, must reflect and embody the commands, obedience, and example of Jesus in dealing with the subjects of medical ethics (and all other subjects). Here, as so often, the meaning of Jesus Christ divided not only Jew from Christian but also Christian from Christian (Lammers 1988).

The scholars who would study what future archaeologists dug up when they found this series in *Second Opinion* would deduce the central issue when a medical ethicist began with or brought up *theos:* What is the character of this Other? All the thinkers recognized that the human situation needed divine address; there is a "fault" (Verhey 1988: 107), a flaw, a need for sustenance and redemption. But the main assertion about God is that God is creator of all people and all things.

If people asserted something like that, as most people in this culture did, there had to be consequences in ethics. For Ramsey, "the world is God's creation, dependent on God for its being, order, and future," and hence, he went on, it served as a base for "establishing the equal worth of all people, whatever their social status." For Ramsey and others, this also meant that the case method was an excellent way of discerning need, for one should make crucial determinants of ethical action on the basis of study "of the historical world, rather than from revelation" (Smith 1987: 112). Gustafson and all the others reasoned that medical ethics acquired a special character when all that is, is perceived as "gift" (Verhey 1988: 118). For all, as with Bernard Häring, the response to creation and gift implies "stewardship," a sense that exacts care and carefulness. Creation is unfinished, and the human — including the researcher, the physician, the cooperating patient, the ethicist — all become "cocreators" (Hamel 1991: 118). Such is the testimony of these unearthed texts.

While all the thinkers set the human in a natural context and cared about the whole created environment, they were especially attentive to humans themselves and, with Häring, could be described in general, though not as members of a technically defined school, as *personalists.* Care for the person, for each person, in generally nonpaternalistic ways, came close to being an obsessive theme in these essays. For Häring, the person outranked even the application of divine law and certainly of human law (Hamel 1991: 112). There must, he argued, be a "resacralization" of the person if the gift of creation was to be properly stewarded.

Grisez, using natural law and Catholic doctrine as his basis for reasoning, was explicit and firm about his point of view: basic goods and human beings "are both incommensurable and nonfungible," that is, "they admit of no common measure enabling us to say that one is more valuable than another. Nor without loss could we replace one basic good with another, or even with another instance of the same sort of good." Commodities like soybeans "are fungible, exchangeable. Babies are not. Nor are friendships or any other of the basic goods." Not all of Grisez's colleagues found the notion of nonexchangeability and non-fungibility to be quite so determinative, but they matched him in concern for the distinctiveness and value of all humans (Hanink 1990: 89-90).

With surprising frequency these thinkers relied on the concept of "covenant," so familiar in Hebrew Scriptures and Reformed Protestant (Calvinist, Puritan) treatises and hence in many American Protestant spheres but less widely used in some other Christian communions. David H. Smith sent up an alert: "The first step in understanding Paul Ramsey's moral theory is to recognize that it is controlled and informed by prior faith commitments: it is covenant-centered. Its basis is the assumption that God has made a covenant with people and that people therefore have an obligation to be faithful to that covenant" (Smith 1987: 108). This covenantal thinking in many of the figures — less so in Childress than in the others — qualified their talk about the "autonomy" of individuals. Here Gustafson was most explicit, as Verhey condensed his position: " 'Certainly it is correct to respect [persons'] capacity for agency,' Gustafson says, 'but persons are more than their capacity for agency. . . . We are to respect persons not merely as individuals but as "members one of another" in their communities'" (Verhey 1988: 108). Germain Grisez, less predictably a covenantal thinker, notes that "all our moral insights are deepened by our covenant relationship with God" (Hanink 1990: 92). William F. May developed the notion most decisively, having written extensively on covenant in the professions and at book length on the physician's covenant (Meilaender 1989: 105). It may impress the future reader that one could write the story of theological ethics in this period as an elaboration of the concepts of divine creation and divine-human relations based on covenant. This combination separated theological ethics from the "contractual" thinking that dominated desacralized and secularized medical ethics.

Another way to put the case for the human side of the covenant is this: Whether through obedience to divine law (Gellman 1991: 100), involvement with the Christian "story" (Lammers 1988: 133), or attention to "deontology," that is, ethics based on duty (Smith 1987: 108), a key characteristic was always "response." Ordinary medical ethics was

252

responsive to the needs of a patient, but theological ethics perceived all creativity, stewardship, care, research, and provision of resources to be part of a response to the divine "Thou" who demanded response — and graciously made it possible, even in a broken world where all actions are partial.

One peculiar stress of a number of these thinkers was on the theme of justice. Who merited care when not all could have care, as in the case of kidney dialysis or heart transplants? Paul Ramsey and James Childress, starting from somewhat different bases, both employed an inelegant but easy to understand coinage: to use Ramsey's term, one "randomized," either through lottery or by priority in line — but not by measuring who merited attention because she or he was of higher value (Smith 1987: 116). And according to Courtney Campbell, "Childress reflects the views of Paul Ramsey in holding that the experience of God's indiscriminate love for human beings provides a morally significant analogy that favors equality in rationing decisions and rules out social worth assessments" (Campbell 1989: 135).

The fact that different thinkers began at different points did not mean that they never converged on their themes and conclusions. For an example of convergence: *community,* in the responsive context of covenantal thinking, was a prime element for most. Hauerwas, naturally, made it central. For him, the community was the church. "Hauerwas thus explicitly counters the individualistic understanding of the person that he finds in modern society. He counters with the church, which for him stands against not only this society but any political society. Unlike modern society, the church is formed by the conviction that God rules the world, and it bears witness to this fact" (Lammers 1988: 137). So persistent and dominant was this theme that Hauerwas's critics claimed that he had little to say about the ethical possibilities of non-Christians. "His response is quite simple: the church is his social ethic" (Lammers 1988: 137).

This is not the place to follow these case-minded personalists through the sample "hard cases" to which almost all of them attended consistently and exemplarily. Not all of them would be relevant in the time of the future archaeologists, thanks to anticipated technological changes that would occasion fresh framing of issues. Few writers in this series could avoid the topic of abortion, perhaps the most controversial issue that emerged in their time. The spectrum of positions was wide, beginning with Grisez on one end, in what might be called a "pure prolife" situation — in code language, not exactly theirs, "better two deaths than one murder" — and moving to much more qualified and tempered treatments across the range of possibilities. Given their presuppositions, including the pervasive wariness most of them showed toward individualism and autonomy, none of them would be on the "pure prochoice" end, which would have meant that nothing but the decision of the isolated woman mattered, that no life issue was at stake. No, for these writers fetal life was also a divine creation, a gift, which demanded response and stewardship in the context of covenant and community.

Similarly, at the other end of the life span, all nine were attentive to issues associated with death. There were distinctives here, too, born of religious faith. As preoccupied with persons as they all were, they did not see the mere extension of biological existence as the only and highest good. Whatever their (generally cautious) stands on euthanasia, many of them stressed that the community-based character of theological ethics made "walking with" the patient the urgent ethical theme. Thus, for Ramsey, when the patient started to die, the talk of *cure* became irrelevant. "Now the most serious problems are discomfort and loneliness. Medical care for the dying instead requires providing *comfort*, that is, symptom control and company" (Smith 1987: 123).

Similarly, for May, "death is not only a crisis of the flesh. It is . . . a crisis of community. . . . Death will also reveal — starkly and unmistakably — something about the communities in which the dying person lives," just as it brings another crisis, of separation from God. May's approach to all this was to give explicit witness to the fact of "death's powerlessness over against the love of God [which] has been revealed and enacted in Jesus. This frees us from the power of death as a sacral reality, frees us from either preoccupation with or avoidance of death" (Meilaender 1989: 111). An ethic of Christian address to Christian was particular here.

In earlier ages the intrusion of God-language into ethical situations usually came down from a human hierarchy and was asserted dogmatically and repressively. Modern medical ethics was born in a time when religious triumphalism had come to be seen as a foolish expression. The address of most of these nine thinkers and their nine expositors tended to be quite modest. May spoke of theological ethics as offering a "corrective view" more than as having all the answers (Meilaender 1989: 112). Regarding what the theological ethicist had to offer, almost all the thinkers shared Gustafson's word: *limited*. As Verhey condensed Gustafson's position, "Theology qualifies the fundamental orientation of a person's life, . . . but it can qualify judgments about conduct only indirectly, only through the process of discernment used to reach them. 'From the standpoint of immediate practicality, the contribution of theology is not great'" (Verhey 1988: 116).

Such a sense of finitude, ignorance, and limitation was appropriate, given the complexities, but all the thinkers acknowledged that issues beyond "immediate practicality" went into the personal relations of the patients' world and that of those who seek well-being. *Discernment* was an often-used term in the calls of these responsive thinkers (Verhey 1988: 108; Hamel 1991: 124; Meilaender 1989: 116). The important issues tended to be settled not only as prime-time and page-one addresses to crises and dilemmas. They had to do with understandings of creation as gift, evoking stewardship; of covenant, involving response; of community, countering autonomous individualism and loneliness. Through all the writings there was evident an awareness that the human condition is, in its own terms, a tragedy (Lammers 1988: 180) not to be overcome by casual or brusque and oversure ethical comment, including or especially by theologians.

At times as one reviews these essays a temptation comes to the reader to ask for less of the "relentless consistency" with which people like Ramsey pursued uncomfortable themes. Here and there one looks for a lighter moment, a grace note to go with the witness to grace, the gift of relief to go with the perduring testimony to gravity. Yet the seriousness of these thinkers, who — as the archaeologists would have found had they had a chance to know them in personal encounter — by and large were good company, *bon vivant* types who loved life as they loved theology and ethics as these related to life, is apparent.

In their seriousness they kept demonstrating a kind of "go slow" approach to ethics when the character and quality of human life were concerned. It has been said that once upon a time when the theologian was too obtrusive and obstructive, the scientist had to serve as the guardian of human freedom. In the period of modern medical ethics, science and technology, even in the most ethical and discerning hands, could be the limiters of human freedom and barriers to community. In such a situation the concerns manifest in the work of these 18 thinkers might well have performed humanizing and personalizing functions both in the communities that shared something of their theistic faiths

255

and those that rejected such faiths outright. The archaeologists of the future who came across these writings would be struck by the authors' genuine interest in seeing the details of bodily and social existence thrown against the background that offered the largest scope. That meant a resort to the concept of God, of *Theos*, as in *theology*. They were ready to speak and write in this manner fully aware of the difficulty induced by God-talk in a society that describes itself as secular and pluralist. The prospect for yield, in their eyes, is too great for them to be content with lesser concepts. They leave a rich legacy for the generations that, though they use different terms, also speak of ethics, the good, and God.

References

Cahill, Lisa Sowle. 1988. "On Richard McCormick: Reason and Faith in Post–Vatican II Catholic Ethics." *Second Opinion* 9 (November): 108-30.

Campbell, Courtney S. 1989. "On James F. Childress: Answering Every Person." *Second Opinion* 11 (July): 118-44.

Davis, Dena. 1991. "Beyond Rabbi Hiyya's Wife: Women's Voices in Jewish Bioethics." *Second Opinion* 16 (March): 10-30.

Gellman, Marc. 1991. "On Immanuel Jakobovits: Bringing the Ancient Word to the Modern World." *Second Opinion* 17, no. 1 (July): 97-117.

Hamel, Ron P. 1991. "On Bernard Häring: Construing Medical Ethics Theologically." *Second Opinion* 17, no. 2 (October): 108-27.

Hanink, James G. 1990. "On Germain Grisez: Can Christian Ethics Give Answers?" *Second Opinion* 15 (November): 84-100.

Lammers, Stephen E. 1988. "On Stanley Hauerwas: Theology, Medical Ethics, and the Church." *Second Opinion* 8 (July): 128-47.

Meilaender, Gilbert. 1989. "On William F. May: Corrected Vision for Medical Ethics." *Second Opinion* 10 (March): 104-24.

Smith, David H. 1987. "On Paul Ramsey: A Covenant-Centered Ethic for Medicine." *Second Opinion* 6 (November): 107-27.

Verhey, Allen D. 1988. "On James M. Gustafson: Can Medical Ethics Be Christian?" *Second Opinion* 7 (March): 104-27.